STRESS RELIEF

for the

ANXIOUS MIND

Practical Advice to
De-Stress Your Life in
5 Minutes a Day

Lauren Ryan

Table of Contents

Introduction

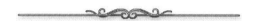

All my life, I was trained to believe that stress results from major life events, such as a death in the family, a change in career, or even the end of a relationship. But stress is also a by-product of ordinary life. Living in a fast-paced society, developing and maintaining healthy coping mechanisms isn't an option - it's a necessary survival skill. If we don't control our stress, it will control us. Without adequate self-care and stress management, we usually push ourselves before crashing for some time. But prolonged exposure to stress has serious physical, mental, and emotional consequences. Too much stress puts the body in continual fight or flight mode. While trying to compensate for the energy it loses, the body depletes its essential resources. As a result, systems begin to shut down over time.

For me, the process was gradual. I didn't fully realize it was happening until one night when I came home from work and basically collapsed onto my couch. It had been a long week of putting in overtime. My husband was working even longer hours back then, and I was responsible for redecorating our brand new condominium. Weekends were for squeezing in social events and time with both sets of parents. I was especially careful to make time for my husband's parents, who were visiting from Florida and eager to spend all the time they could with us.

I guess you could say that I was functioning on autopilot through my days. On the surface, I finally had everything I'd dreamed of and worked hard for all my life: a loving husband, a dream house, and a burgeoning career I hoped would take us places - preferably on some well-deserved tropical vacation!

But it looked as though this was never going to happen. No matter how many hours of overtime I put in, more work seemed to pile up. Sometimes, my schedule was so heavy that I had nightmares about being the victim of a terrible car accident. In my worst nightmares, I was lying underneath a pileup of cars. In order to get up, I'd have to push them off, which is impossible. It didn't take me long to understand that this recurring dream was a metaphor for my rising stress levels. I really did feel like the woman in that nightmare. That's how little freedom I had over my life and the choices I made on a daily basis.

It got to the point where I didn't know what was wrong with me. By all accounts, I had what appeared to be "the perfect life". I thought I must be weak or even unappreciative of what I had. But on the night I came home from work and found myself so tired I could barely move, I was forced to ask myself some important questions. How much was I actually enjoying the life I had created? My husband and I hardly saw each other, even though we lived in the same house.

We were working so hard, yet we still didn't have the money to take time off and do the things we'd envisioned by this age. Everywhere I looked on social media, I was inundated with images of thirty-somethings expanding their horizons, traveling to new countries and exploring new terrain. It seemed that so many things I wanted loomed just out of reach. It was an endless cycle. I told myself, "Lauren, if you just work a little more, push yourself a little harder, your dreams will start to come to fruition!"

But saving money was hard with our new mortgage, and my husband and I had to work almost constantly just to afford our new place. Actually, the adorable condominium I had fallen in love with at first sight was quickly becoming another source of stress. It was a fixer upper, but seemed so full of promise. I hadn't realized how endless the remodeling and redecorating process would be.

The bottom line is, most of what I did during my day was for others. I was expending so much energy externally that there was nothing left to nurture my inner self. I had lost touch with many of my own wants and needs. In fact, I felt so disconnected from myself that I began to wonder if being numbed by routine was what adult life was all about - the price people pay for having a home, a career, a relationship. A life. Where had I gone wrong?

A sense of loneliness and isolation engulfed me as I sat on the couch. I knew my husband was upstairs in his office, catching up on some work. But somehow, I couldn't even bring myself to get up and start dinner. I just felt so burned out. My energy core was utterly depleted, and it wasn't regenerating the way it used to. I was always able to somehow force myself to get up and go, but inside I was drained of the joy and motivation I used to bring to work and relationships. My nerves were stretched so tight and thin that I was honestly afraid I'd just snap. I had the overwhelming sensation that my life was held together by a thread. The gap between the woman I was and the woman I wanted to be was growing. My dreams felt far from reality.

Was it like this for everyone, or was it just me?

This was a question to which I spent several months searching for an answer. I made a promise to myself that I was going take control of my life again. As I researched stress, I learned more about its physiological and psychological causes and manifestations. The body and mind are more interconnected than most of us fully understand. Learning about the ways in which my own body and mind influence each other was a real lifesaver.

I also realized that there are unique components to living and working in today's modern world. Technology has expanded many of the industries we work in, adding endless new opportunities. The flipside is that our work environments are also complicated by pressures and demands. Industries may be expanding, but costs are also rising for the average adult. I'm sure I don't need to make a PSA here, but it has never been more expensive to afford a home, pay daily living expenses, and repay education loans. In fact, many of us are in considerable debt before we even start our lives, so we don't have a clean slate to begin with. Most of us are fighting for places in the competitive job market. This dog-eat dog mentality has become a cornerstone of our society. There's a tendency to prioritize work over health, self-care and meaningful relationships.

Add parenthood to this list, and your plate isn't just too full - it's spilling over!

I knew that restoring my health and happiness involved changing my thought patterns, and that I'd have to learn to replace the old with the new. For example, I had the habit of resorting to catastrophic thinking when one thing went wrong; if I encountered a problem with my health or work life, I'd imagine the very worst and convince myself that my entire life was unfolding before my eyes. Every small pain could be cancer; an unexpected disappointment at work could lead to a chain of events that would ruin everything I had worked for. I learned that cognitive behavioral therapy teaches you to strategically replace negative thoughts and behaviors with positive ones, until healthy ways of coping become an ingrained habit.

Although some people find cognitive behavioral therapy extremely helpful, you don't always have to go into therapy to learn how to manage stress well. This book is an in-depth guide to stress management that should help you identify your stressors and the stress management skills that work best for *you*).

In this book, I'll discuss stress management in-depth. I will guide you step-by-step through the process of identifying your stressors, reducing anxiety and replacing unhealthy coping mechanisms with healthy ones. The emphasis is on the term, step-by-step. This book starts with baby steps toward stress reduction and implanting self-care into your routine. I understand that this is a process, so my goal is to give you the tools you need to prepare for long-term success. I know from experience that it isn't easy to change the way you respond to stress, so we'll start with ways you can reduce its harmful effects in just five minutes a day.

But the most important concept I want you to understand is that in order for this book to help you, you have to commit to making a change. The most important commitment you'll ever make is to yourself. (Yes, that applies to parents, too! As primary caregivers, you owe it to yourself and to your kids to be the happiest, healthiest version of you that you can be). Stress is a universal struggle, and we all owe it to ourselves to make room for change and growth.

We owe it to ourselves to avoid triggers and toxic environments and to handle stress in the healthiest way possible. I wrote this book to provide you with the knowledge and strength to do this. Like me, you might feel that the stress in your life controls your feelings, daily habits and major decisions. But believe it or not, you have the power to make changes so you can control your stress, and not the other way around. I realize that everyone who reads this book has his or her own unique set of stressors, and I am going to cover as many of them as possible. I'm a firm believer that there is immense power and strength in numbers. We've got to help each other - and receive help - if we want to be the best possible versions of ourselves. People are naturally interdependent; our energies and stress levels are connected by the way we treat and influence one another.

But remember: Your health and happiness ultimately depend on your willingness to make a commitment to yourself. Do it here and now: make a promise to yourself to change the way you relate to your body and mind in the presence of stressors. My hope is that opening this book will reveal a new world of possibilities, and a new, happier life.

Wait! Before You Start...

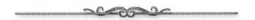

I know you're anxious to get reading, but before you do I wanted to tell you about a free companion resource for this book.

As you'll find out in Chapter 4, keeping track of your stress levels, through regular weekly check-ins, is a great way to keep track of your progress and increase your awareness of stress in your life. But there's also evidence that your stress levels can improve just by taking the time to track them!

I've put together a stress self-assessment worksheet to make analyzing your personal stress levels easy (and maybe even fun). Simply fill out the 10 question worksheet to find out your Stress Score. Then repeat the test every week (it only takes a few minutes) and you'll gain insight and awareness into your stress levels and how they are progressing. Plus, you get to watch your scores improve as you make your way through the book.

You can download the worksheet on my website here:

https://www.bcfpublishing.com/stress-assessment

I don't want you to have to wait until Chapter 4 to get this benefit, so download the worksheet and get started tracking your scores today.

1

Understanding

"The well bred contradict other people.
The wise contradict themselves."

– Oscar Wilde

To combat stress, you have to understand it. There are various ways you can try to cope, including classes that teach you coping skills, medications that reduce stress hormones, or cognitive behavioral therapy. That said, even if you do any of these things, if you don't really understand stress, why it happens, how it works, etc., you will never be able to prevail. Although you may have a general idea of what stress looks like, such that you know how to identify it, you also need to understand the mechanisms behind it.

Stress is a biological mechanism designed to protect the body. Specifically, it's a chemical reaction that your brain sends, telling your body how to react to protect itself. These chemical "stress signals" trigger a specific process that enables you to fight, flee, or defend yourself. The key here is that you can't carry out any of the self-preservation methods if you haven't first identified the stressor. Clearly, there are countless types of stress, and just as many reactions, but the chemical reaction within the body is the same for every individual.

Stress is not completely avoidable, nor should it be. By its very nature, the feeling of stress is a protective mechanism. If you don't know something is bothering you or potentially dangerous, you can't react accordingly. Consider the analogy of a child touching a hot stove. He touches the stove and jerks his head back because he got burned. That's a form of stress. The brain immediately sends a signal warning the child that the extreme heat is dangerous, so he pulls away. Some people have a medical condition that prevents them from feeling pain, and children with that condition are in grave danger because they literally don't feel anything when they get cut, bruised, bumped, burned, etc., so they don't seek help from their parents. Luckily, there is no illness that prevents humans from feeling stress. It's a necessary biological signal, however much we may not enjoy it, and once you understand it, you can learn to deal with it.

WHAT IS STRESS

Stress is a response to a threat of danger. When you perceive that something bad might happen, whether it actually will or not, your body readies itself to be combative and resolving in order to overcome the stressor. If you feel as though a basic human need might be taken away or just something that brings you pleasure, you are going to feel stressed out. When you fear that something dangerous is about to happen, or if you have work you don't know how you are going to complete, you will start to feel the effects of stress.

It the famous fight-or-flight response. When presented with any sort of threat, either you will feel the need to face it and fight it off, or you become scared and run. In either scenario, the body needs the proper tools to react. If you are going to fight the threat, you need the energy to be strong, so that it does not overcome you. If you feel the need to run, you have to make sure that you are strong enough to outrun the threat and handle yourself. This is common in all animals, not just humans, and applies to all ages as well.

It is automatic preparation for a future harmful situation. Bodies are built to protect themselves, which is why they have specific parts and reactions, different chemicals and varied responses dependent on one's background, religion, lifestyle, and genetic makeup. What is absolutely true for all, however, is that everyone experiences stress based on a perceived threat. These threats present themselves in different ways, but it will always remain true that you will become stressed out when threatened.

It sounds a little strange to put it in this context. When you are standing in line at a restaurant and learn that they are out of a certain ingredient, you might feel a pang of stress, wondering what you are going to order. You don't feel inherently threatened, but your body doesn't know the difference when you feel a little stressed out, so you react in the same way.

The Chemicals Involved

The chemical process that triggers stress begins with the release of cortisol. Cortisol is a steroid hormone produced by the adrenal glands, leading you to feel the flight-or-fight sensation. Biologically speaking, this surge of cortisol causes you to feel momentarily stronger or faster than you usually are, allowing for those made-for-TV moments; for instance, when a person can pry a heavy object off a loved one, because of the temporary adrenal rush. More prosaically, the release of cortisol may cause you to be more focused, alert, and ready to address whatever danger has activated your stress hormone.

Beyond helping you cope with stressful situations, cortisol also plays a key role in digestion. Your body requires glucose as a source of ready energy, and cortisol regulates glucose production. As long as you're stressed, this hormone will be produced, and so will higher levels than normal of glucose. Research has shown that high levels of cortisol (read: stress) can lead to weight gain, because of the overabundance of glucose (sugar).

Aside from weight gain, high levels of cortisol can affect memory. That's ironic, given that at the outset when first released, it leads to that hyperfocused, alert state mentioned earlier. But this can only last so long before your brain becomes exhausted. The fact is, you only need a certain amount of cortisol, and when too much is released, it has negative effects, including some that can be deadly.

Clearly, you want to minimize your stress levels both for your personal comfort and to remain healthy. You don't want to tax your energy reserves at unnecessary moments. Imagine that you had the terrible day described earlier, were stressed out nonstop, and then you had to deal with a real emergency at the end of the day. You've already expended many of your physical, emotional and mental resources. You won't be able to deal with the situation nearly as well as you would have had you not been stressed the entire day.

Adolescents are especially affected by high levels of cortisol. Given that their brains are still developing, a consistent rush of cortisol can weaken their organ systems and affect their overall development, including brain structure. This can cause mental health issues, learning problems, etc. Thus, children need to be taught how to deal with stress as much as adults.

Looking to the Past

How you were raised and the environment in which you grew up have affected you. Everybody knows that. But not everybody focuses on how your biology might have been impacted by childhood. As mentioned, kids continually subjected to stress are impacted even more than adults, and on multiple levels. Furthermore, those kids grow up to be adults, who may not know how to cope with stress in a healthy manner. Children naturally develop survival skills that they often don't transfer to the adult world. For example, an abused child might deal with stress by learning to avoid personal relationships. As an adult, it's less likely that such a person will be able to hide in a room all day to get away from people who might potentially hurt him or her. Therefore, that adult will be perpetually stressed when surrounded by people, afraid of being hurt again and not know how to deal with the constant fear.

Another example of childhood stress is comfort eating. If you were subjected to constant stress, maybe you turned to food to escape. As an adult, you might still be using that same stress-escape mechanism, only now it's beginning to cause problems beyond weight gain. Maybe your heart is being affected. Your cholesterol. Your mobility to and from work.

You need a better way of dealing with normal, everyday stress, but you haven't learned it yet.

Some people handle stress better than others. That's a basic fact. And it's probably rooted in how one learns to cope as a child. If, when carrying a heavy high school workload, a teenager is advised how best organize his time and efforts and learns how to prioritize, that teenager will probably do a good job as an adult when it comes to handling the countless everyday tasks in an office, for example. An adult who didn't learn basic skills can be overwhelmed when he or she now has to do ten different assignments in a day and, as a result, may be constantly stressed.

If some people seem stressed all the time, it's probably because they are. They view the world as a stressful place, because that was how they first perceived it as kids. Although stress can have positive aspects, people subjected to it since childhood may not be able to see anything but the negative. Then, it becomes a cycle: *this happened, it was bad, I'm unhappy and worried, so then the next thing that happens also seems terrible, and now I'm even more unhappy and worried*, and on and on.

Your brain likes routine. As such, it excels at establishing patterns of behavior. You may have heard that once you repeat something seven times, it becomes a habit. That's how your brain works. When you do something over and over, whether it's always brushing your teeth before bed or checking both ways before crossing the street, your brain is trained to follow that particular behavior pattern and thought. Similarly, when you train your brain as a child to react to stress in a certain way, it carries into adulthood. If you learned to laugh at stress, you might be that adult who can shrug off a terrible, no good, really bad day. But if you learned to get angry or tearful the moment stress hit, you could be that adult who explodes the moment a small crisis presents itself at work or in his personal life.

Children naturally mimic their elders. You undoubtedly learned some of your stress-coping skills from the adults around you. If your father came home from work and always threw his bag across the room because he was so frustrated, as an adult, you might aggressively drop books or papers on your work desk, for instance. If your mom slammed doors angrily, you might do the same in a misguided attempt to cope with stress.

In the *Biological Psychiatry Journal*, a study of Holocaust survivors finds that there are similar genetic alterations in the same places in the brains of both parents and children. "This is the first demonstration of an association of preconception parental trauma with epigenetic alterations that is evident in both exposed parent and offspring, providing potential insight into how severe psychophysiological trauma can have intergenerational effects" (Yehuda, Daskalakis, Bierer, Bader, et al., 2016). The study suggests that stress can literally rewire the brain to the point where the way you react likely has a genetic link to how an ancestor once coped. This doesn't mean that habits can't be changed; but it does make clear that reactions to stress are sometimes coded at the genetic level, explaining why it is very hard for some individuals to face with stress, while others just let it roll off their backs.

Evolutionary Purpose of Stress

As noted, stress is a biological mechanism designed to protect the self. Just as you walk through a bad day in the twenty-first century, consider a bad day during the Stone Age. You wake up one morning in your cave, only to find that someone slipped in while you were sleeping and stole every bit of meat from a hunt a couple days' back. It's snowing, so the chances of getting another kill are unlikely. You may be hungry for a while. Then you walk out of your cave and realize that the river close by has flooded, and you have to rush to higher ground. While you're literally running for your life, you encounter a predator and have to run in the opposite direction to keep from becoming its dinner. You manage to survive, but night comes and you don't have a new cave. The wood is soggy and you can't start a fire. Your stomach is growling. You don't dare close your eyes because you're completely exposed to the elements and any animals or unfriendly fellow cavemen. You don't know the first thing about science, but cortisol helps you stay awake and alert in spite of your hunger and exhaustion until day dawns and you find a safe place to finally get some rest. You live another day, and as a result, you may have a chance of finding a mate and reproducing, thereby passing on your genes—and in those genes, the hardwired survival mechanism so ingrained in you.

The above may sound comical, but it's not intended to be. All of those things undoubtedly happened to your ancestors at some point, and they had to learn to cope with literal life-threatening stress. Who knows how they did it? Maybe they threw rocks in frustration. The point is, human bodies evolved to cope with stress. But back then, it was often—maybe almost always—life or death related. Nowadays, the stresses faced are not nearly as dangerous. So you can't flag a taxi down in the pouring rain. You won't die. So you burned dinner. You won't die. You locked your key in the car. You won't die. Nevertheless, you still have to cope. Unfortunately, the cortisol that kept your caveman ancestor awake all night might also be keeping you in the twenty-first century. But he had to watch for bears. What are you watching for when awake all night? Bills? That long-delayed promotion? A fight you just had with a friend? While it was useful for the caveman to remain awake, you won't solve any conflicts by staying awake all night. And yet. You do.

Your body is still trying to protect you, just as it has evolved to do. In this case, the bear is something less tangible, but still something your brain feels you need cortisol to deal with. While, of course, you sometimes do deal with literal danger in your day-to-day world, for the most part, you're not going to be physically hurt by whatever conflict you're facing, whether internal or external. Nevertheless, your ingrained biology won't give you a pass, regardless of the situation. Why?

Survival. Your body still wants you to survive so you can reproduce and pass on your genes. Ironically, the stress hormones designed to protect you can also literally kill you. Many studies show that death rates rise in the immediate aftermath of major life events like divorce or a loved one's passing. While, back in the day, having all those stress hormones might have helped you elude a predator, nowadays they usually just lead to heart attacks, strokes, and any number of other stress-related ailments.

Now you need new coping tools. Ones appropriate for the here-and-now rather than for a caveman. You need to learn strategies to deal with stress, so you get immediate relief and prevent the toxic accumulation of cortisol, along with a whole host of negative side effects. The aim of this book is to help you find the necessary stress relief, both for your mental and physical health.

HOW STRESS IS CREATED IN YOUR BRAIN

You know all too well what causes external stress. But what causes the specific chemical reaction inside that triggers the fight-or-flight syndrome? You can look at it like a game of telephone happening inside your body. The message gets passed from place to place, and, eventually, the message becomes distorted.

Stress starts in your amygdala, at the base of your brain. This walnut-sizes brain structure is sometimes referred to as "the fear center." Research has shown that people who feel constant fear have large amygdalae. When the amygdala senses a danger, it sends a signal to the hypothalamus.

The hypothalamus is kind of like a cockpit that radios commands. When the amygdala's signal reaches the hypothalamus, this organ, in turn, contacts your body's autonomic nervous system (ANS). The ANS controls major bodily functions like breathing and heartbeat. It is divided into the brain and spinal cord in one section, and the parasympathetic nervous system (PNS) and the sympathetic nervous system (SNS) in another.

The SNS is what causes the physical fight or flight reaction. When danger arises, the SNS tells the adrenal glands to release cortisol and adrenaline. In combination, these hormones make your heart race, causing you to breathe faster, sending blood rushing from your arms and legs to vital organs, so you feel like your fingertips are numb, for instance (as in the case of a panic attack), and triggering the release of glucose in your digestive system, among other events in a massive biological chain reaction.

In this game of telephone, maybe you were spooked when you thought someone was following you down the street. You weren't, but the fear you felt was erroneously passed down along the chain of communication, becoming magnified at each place, until you hyperventilated and trembled for no reason. The system worked like it was supposed to, trying to protect you, but ultimately it just stressed you more and taxed your energy for no reason at all.

After the stressful event passes—in this case, after you realize you're not being followed while walking home—the PNS takes over and acts as a kind of depressant, easing the brain's foot off the gas pedal, if you will, and allowing you to gradually relax once more.

How Your Body Reacts to Stress

Now you understand how your brain reacts to stress. But what about your body? Well, stress affects every single part, starting with your musculoskeletal system. When you're stressed, do your shoulders hunch up? Pay attention next time you're dealing with a conflict. Very likely, they do. Does your head ache? That's also likely. What about your stomach? Do you feel tension in your abs? Could be. That's all because the muscles in your body tense up in reaction to a stressor. They're trying to prepare you to either turn around and defend yourself, or to spring forward and run for your life as fast as you can.

Next, your respiratory system is affected. When the hypothalamus communicates with the ANS and adrenaline is released, your lungs open wider. Your body is trying to help you get plenty of oxygen during a crisis, so you don't pass out. That extra oxygen can also help you focus more in a tense situation. That's why you might find yourself panting when you're afraid; it's your body's biological reaction to stress. However, if you hyperventilate—breathe too fast— for too long, the opposite of what your body wants will occur; you'll get lightheaded and dizzy. (Think of a person having a panic attack, needing to breathe into a paper bag.) That's because your body's stress reaction is meant to be short and controlled, not un- limited.

Your muscles, then your lungs…next is your cardiovascular system, your heart. This is the part of the body that most people understand is impacted by stress. When your amygdala triggers a stress signal, your blood vessels dilate to allow blood to flow through more rapidly, and your heart starts pounding to push that blood through. It's yet another biological reaction designed to give you the strength to get you out of danger as fast as possible.

After the heart, comes the gastrointestinal system. Stress can cause a drop in blood flow or oxygen to the system. The reasons for this aren't entirely clear, but it's possible that the body may be trying to prevent the spread of toxins, and the gastrointestinal system is in large part responsible for carrying substances around the body. The lower blood flow and lack of oxygen can cause cramps, ulcers, or diarrhea. Connected to your stomach, your esophagus will also be affected if bile backs up into it, causing stress-related heartburn.

Stress is still moving through your body. Now your reproductive system is impacted. As a woman, if you're constantly stressed, your body may try to defend you by stopping your periods. Your sexual desire may be affected, because your body doesn't want you reproducing when you're in poor physical shape. If you're pregnant, stress might cause you to miscarry. If you're not pregnant, stress may make it difficult to conceive. If you're a man, stress can impact your stress production and/or testosterone levels (directly connected to sexual desire.) All of this, again, is just your body trying to defend you. If you're under attack, you shouldn't be reproducing, and your body is doing its best to stop that from happening.

So, from head to toe, stress impacts your entire body. If stress is limited in duration, there won't be long-term effects. But imagine all of the above happening for extended periods of time, and it's pretty easy to see why the effects will be less than salutary.

Long-Term Health Effects of Stress

Let's run down the list of effects on the body mentioned above, but focusing more on long-term physical impacts.

The musculoskeletal system

A chronically-stressed person, who is suffering from perpetually tight muscles, might develop anything from constant neck, back, and shoulder problems to issues with tendons and ligaments and brittle bones. Yes. Stress is believed to cause difficulty with some vitamin absorption, which can lead to weakened bones. Because of all the muscular tension, migraines can develop.

The respiratory system

Chronically-stressed people are more prone to conditions like asthma and chronic obstructive pulmonary disease (COPD.) A weakened immune system can also leave a stressed person vulnerable to pneumonia and the flu.

The cardiovascular system

Heart attacks, strokes, thickened arteries, and malfunctioning heart valves—these are just a few of the ways that the cardiovascular system can be impacted by constant stress.

The gastrointestinal system

As said earlier, cramps, ulcers, and diarrhea can be directly related to stress. Other negative effects that stress has on the gastrointestinal system include kidney stones or gallstones, irritable bowel syndrome (IBS), and gastroesophageal reflux disease (GERD).

The reproductive system

In addition to all the ill effects that stress brings to the reproductive system, other possible stress effects include polycystic ovarian syndrome, hot flashes, and difficulty achieving or maintaining an erection.

EFFECTS OF STRESS ON MOOD

All of these physical problems start in the brain, which sends out the initial stress signal. Of course, the brain itself is directly affected and chronic stress has a terrible impact on a person's mental health and mood. Chronic stress, it has been shown, can affect the chemicals that regulate brain function. "Feel good" hormones like serotonin may be suppressed by constant stress. This can lead to things like depression or exacerbate conditions like bipolar disorder.

Chronic stress can affect your focus, discussed earlier. If you're concentrating constantly on just surviving/getting through the day, this leaves you very little energy to focus on more important matters. You might start to feel so exhausted that you become detached from reality or removed from a situation. That's your brain giving you a chance to rest.

Anger is another common reaction to constant stress. It makes sense—your body is in constant survival mode, with every single physical resource taxed. This doesn't leave much room for a person to cope with the little irritants that crop up in our daily lives. Eventually, something as simple as a missing stapler might cause you to explode, because your emotional resources are stretched too thin. Your tight muscles are aching, your heart is pounding, you're hyperventilating, your stomach hurts, and you have heartburn…any person constantly feeling even a few of these symptoms is bound to be in a foul mood.

Anxiety

When your brain is constantly under stress, it reacts by trying to find ways to cope. Unfortunately, these ways are usually hardwired to help you deal with purported dangers, so your stress is only further exacerbated. Simply put: if your brain feels like you are in constant danger, then it's going to make sure you feel constantly anxious and afraid in order to make sure you stay on your guard and remain safe.

According to the Mayo Clinic, stress-related anxiety disorders may include, among others:

- Panic attacks
- Social anxiety disorder (fear of socializing)

- Selective mutism (usually seen in children—a refusal to speak in certain situations)
- Specific phobias (such as acrophobia, claustrophobia, and agoraphobia)

All of these disorders are seen as a result of focusing on the wrong thing. As discussed earlier, the release of cortisol temporarily helps you focus better. It makes you hyperalert. In the case of panic attacks, your brain thinks you're in danger, so it causes you to focus on that particular danger and hyperventilate, tense, and prepare to run or fight. In the case of social anxiety disorder, your brain insists that people are dangerous and tells you to stay from them. Selectively mute children feel constantly endangered and focus obsessively on the safety that silence affords. People with specific phobias are channeling all their stress into one thing in order to cope with a kind of stress so vast that it's safer to address just one element, rather than try to deal with an overwhelming, amorphous feeling of insecurity.

Restlessness

When you're under constant stress, your levels of GABA are reduced and your levels of glutamate increase. GABA is a neurotransmitter that blocks signals in between nerve cells. If your GABA is too low, you may feel depressed. Glutamate, on the other hand, is what's called an "excitatory" neurotransmitter. If there's too much of it, you can have ADHD symptoms, seizures, and something called Restless Leg Syndrome where your legs literally can't stay still. They're always twitching, to the point where you're in pain and exhausted.

It stands to reason that if you're always afraid and on edge, staying still will be difficult because your brain is constantly sending you signals, telling you to keep moving. This might mean that, when you're in a meeting, your feet are constantly tapping, your finger are drumming on a table, or your eyes might even twitch. You're in a state of constant alertness, ready to run, even though there's nothing to run from.

One place where you'll particularly feel the impact of such restlessness is when you try to sleep at night. Think about it. If, during the day, when you actually have things to do to keep you busy, you still feel restive, how much worse is it when you're lying down, trying to relax, attempting to shut your racing thoughts off so you can get some shuteye? Sleep patterns are one of the first things impacted by chronic stress, and a lack of sleep is, in itself, a kind of stress, so it only perpetuates the problem: the less you sleep, the more stressed you are, the more restless you will be, and the more tired you become, and yet you still can't sleep.

Lack of Motivation and Focus

When you're constantly stressed, as noted, your body focuses on the wrong thing. Rather than the big picture, it zeroes in on minutiae like the constant fear of losing your job, even if everything at work seems to be going well. But if you've developed a chronic obsession with not being sure you'll have a job tomorrow, whether or not it's grounded in reality, then you're going to be thinking about that incessantly and will therefore neglect other things. The irony is that, while chronic stress can very definitely help you focus, that focus can be so single-minded that you lose touch with everything else.

Imagine that you're afraid of losing your job. For whatever reason, it's become a permanent, constant fear. You think about it all day long, from the moment you wake up. When you're supposed to be taking notes in a meeting, your mind wanders off to worry about your job, so you miss key parts of the presentation you're supposed to be documenting. When typing up a report, you're still thinking about your job, so you do a sloppy job, miss some key details, and turn in an incomplete assignment. You're so focused on not getting fired that you've lost focus on all the things you could do to keep this from happening.

As noted, chronic stress is deeply wearying and, eventually, you're bound to lose motivation. *Well,* you think, *if I'm going to lose my job, I might as well not even try anymore.* This lack of motivation may then turn into a self-fulfilling prophecy where you actually do lose your job, because you were focused on the wrong things and unmotivated when it came to doing what you were hired to do.

This applies to other situations, such as a relationship, for instance. If all you're doing is focusing on the bad things your spouse does, and you're neglecting the bigger picture such as why he's doing them (or how these things are very small compared to all the nice things he does), you're heading for rough waters. And, then, if you feel so defeated that you lose motivation and stop trying, that's even worse. Stress counteractively causes you to lose focus and motivation because your mind is on all the wrong things.

Feeling Overwhelmed

Maybe your stress started with a small incident, like a passing comment your boss made about something you did wrong. That scared you enough that you blew it up out of all proportion and are now obsessing constantly about your job security. Every single day, you come in to work and worry whether it will be your last. You won't be able to pay your bills. You'll lose your house. You'll be humiliated in front of family and friends. You'll never be hired by another company. You'll end up broke, living on someone's couch…

Such a cascade of negative thoughts is as irrational as it is utterly overwhelming. The word "cascade" is apt because, when you're standing under a thundering waterfall, all you feel is the pressure of the water. You don't notice the rocks behind it or the pool below. Your focus is on what is immediately bearing down on you. As a result, if you take a step too far to the left, and are blinded by the spray, you may fall into a very deep pool and drown. In the case of your job, drowning may equate to being fired because you couldn't get past the feel of being utterly overwhelmed.

Life's everyday stresses can certainly be overwhelming. Bills, relationships, medical matters -- you name it. If you don't take them one at a time, it's like walking under a powerful waterfall. Unless trained to do so, your brain will try to take on everything at once, and that's impossible, so you eventually go over the edge.

Irritability and Anger

When you're stressed, you're often angry. More than that, you're irritable. It makes sense. Go back to that feeling of restlessness discussed earlier. You can't sit still. You want to constantly pace. Your body won't allow you to unwind long enough to unclench your muscles. Your head aches. With all the stress you're carrying, of course, you're going to react poorly to additional small stressors.

Let's return to the job stressor scenario. You're worried about that comment your boss made. But you also had a fight with your wife. Plus, the mortgage is due next week, but your bank account is empty. Your kid got in trouble at school. The doctor called and said you need to call her back, urgently.

With all these things weighing on you, a coworker mistakes your lunch in the fridge for hers and opens it. She doesn't eat it. She's just peering into the bag when you walk into the lunchroom. What is your reaction?

If you explode, is it any surprise? Being chronically stressed is just too much. It's too much for your overtaxed body. And it's definitely too much for your constantly stressed mood and mind.

Sadness and Depression

In the midst of the constant, chronic stress some people are under, there are also individuals who are already suffer from mental health issues such as depression. If such a condition already exists, depression is absolutely going to exacerbate it. If the condition *doesn't* already exist, depression just might trigger it due to the chemical imbalance caused by constant stress.

Let's look at sadness . You're having a really rough time. Your salary isn't quite enough to cover your bills. You're always worried that one little incident could happen, and you'll have to dip into your meager savings. Your elderly parents require more and more of your attention, and your husband is feeling neglected. You're butting heads with a coworker.

You have a cold that just won't go away after six weeks. Then the roof starts to leak. Is it any wonder you feel deeply, desperately sad? That sadness is the result of the chronic stress you're under. But what differentiates it from depression?

Sadness has a concrete cause. Depression doesn't always. You might actually be doing quite well. Life is good. And then, for no reason, you wake up and are grief-stricken. You want to cry constantly. Getting out of bed might be almost impossible. Food starts tasting completely bland. You look at yourself in the mirror and hate everything you see, including parts of yourself you used to admire. You might feel yourself going numb, where nothing feels like it matters anymore.

Symptoms like these are hard enough to cope with when there's a reason for them. But when they seem to come out of nowhere, it's even harder, especially when people look at you and say, "But your life is so great!" And you can't help but agree that, yes, it is. But nevertheless, you are suddenly deeply depressed.

Of course, depression does have a cause, even if it doesn't seems to. And very frequently, particularly for people already at risk for depression because of personal trauma or genetic ties to those who have also suffered from depression, stress can be the cause. If you feel some of the following symptoms, listed by the Mayo Clinic, it's very possible you're suffering from major depressive disorder:

- Tearfulness, hopelessness
- Irritability, angry outbursts
- Loss of appetite
- Sleep disturbances—sleeping too much or too little
- Random aches and pains with no explanation
- Difficulty focusing
- Agitation
- Loss of enjoyment of things you used to love
- Fixation on failures/feelings of guilt and personal blame
- Desire to isolate yourself from friends and family

If you are constantly stressed and feeling depressed, be aware that the stress might have triggered a latent depression while also exacerbating your symptoms. Your brain is trying to protect you, but by keeping you constantly on edge in the face of stressful situations, your brain chemistry becomes disrupted and is no longer able to regulate your mood naturally. It's crucial that you seek help from a doctor.

EFFECTS OF STRESS ON BEHAVIOR

As much as stress affects your mind and body, it's bound to also affect your behavior. That, after all, is really your amygdala's goal when it first signals your hypothalamus that there's a problem—the amygdala wants to trigger a behavioral response to an inherent danger. If a caveman constantly sees bears in a certain area, the amygdala puts that man on edge so that he, hopefully, avoids walking back into a place where there's life-threatening danger. Similarly, the amygdala's purpose in the twenty-first century continues to be to keep us safe (and alive).

In short, stress directly affects behavior. Not necessarily in a positive way, mind you, because, as discussed, threats nowadays are rarely life-threatening, and the amygdala may misguidedly try to protect you from something innocuous by erroneously retraining your brain.

Eating Disorders

One stressor that likely didn't exist during the Stone Age was an eating disorder. Back then, you ate and survived or you didn't, and you died. End of story. Nowadays, things are very different.

Modern-day life can be so busy and overwhelming that you look for things to focus on you can control, when everything else is out of your hands. Once such thing is food.

A person who constantly feels like nothing is going right is going to look for the one thing that one hundred percent will ensure control. How much to eat, what to eat, when to eat—these are all highly controllable things. Thus, an overly stressed person might develop an eating disorder. The three major disorders are anorexia, bulimia, and binge eating.

Anorexia

Anorexia, a refusal to eat, often develops in childhood, frequently in children seeking control due to stressors that seem out of their hands. It's very easy to count calories and restrict meal portions. Controlling hunger becomes a challenge that can be "won." Being able to see the numbers on the scale shrink and your clothes loosen is a concrete, tangible feeling of victory for individuals looking for any kind of positive reinforcement.

While it frequently starts in childhood, anorexia can strike at any age. Those most vulnerable are often individuals overwhelmed by problems, who are misguidedly redirecting their anxiety and stress into exerting a death grip over their meals. For someone already slightly insecure about weight, struggling to cope with life's challenges in general, a simple comment such as, "Gee, that shirt looks a little tighter than it used to" can be trigger full-blown anorexia. Although anorexia has a terrible physical impact on the body, it first develops in the brain. In fact, the *Journal of Psychiatry Research: Neuroimaging* published a study documenting enlarged amygdalae in anorexia patients (Joos, Saum, van Elst, et al., 2011).

Bulimia

Bulimia is an eating disorder characterized by binging and purging. Bulimics stuff themselves with huge quantities of food and then force themselves to vomit, sometimes so forcefully that the esophagus ruptures. Similar to anorexia, bulimia very often starts in childhood and is frequently the result of a child trying to find some measure of control. What is more controlling than forcing food down and then forcing it back up?

The journal, *Encephale,* published a research study documenting that "stressful events 65%, anxiety (74%), 'being under pressure' or irritated (51% and 55%) are...major triggers in a majority of the patients" (Rigaud, Jiang, Pennacchio, et al., 2014). Again, there is evidence that stress is a trigger for eating disorders. Vulnerable individuals who already have underlying depressive disorders may be particularly at risk for stress-induced eating disorders such as bulimia.

Binge Eating

Binge eating is considered the most common eating disorder in the United States. It doesn't involve starvation or vomiting but rather involves eating massive quantities of food at least once a week, followed by feelings of abject humiliation and guilt. Why do people do it? In this case, it's more for comfort than control. A child or adult under severe stress may reach for something to soothe him. Food is usually easy to obtain. If so, an individual will gorge herself in an attempt to feel better. The world may be an overwhelming place, full of stressors, but for the few minutes it takes to stuff down the contents of a freezer, things feels a little less unmanageable.

When cortisol is released due to stress, it causes the body to seek out sources of energy in order to flee. The body releases glucose due to cortisol, yes, but if a ready source of calories (energy) is nearby, the brain will trigger a person to seek that, which may very well cause binge eating. A study published in *Appetite* hypothesizes that "cortisol secretion, a major component of the stress response, could play a role in binge eating" (Gluck, 2006).

Anger Outbursts

Just as the amygdala triggers the release of adrenaline and cortisol when you're afraid, when stress makes you angry, a chemical reaction also takes place. As your musculoskeletal system tenses up, chemicals called catecholamines are released. Similar to adrenaline, they make you feel briefly energized, hyperfocused, and strong. Imagine a bottle of soda that's shaken. If the cap is still on, the pressure builds and builds until there's an explosion. Similarly, when you get an infusion of catecholamines due to stress, your body becomes the soda bottle. All those chemicals are flooding through your bloodstream, causing you to feel like you're going to burst. And eventually you do, whether it's shouting, punching, or kicking something, etc.

Earlier, it was noted that constant exposure to cortisol, a stress hormone, has been proven to change brain chemistry and structure. Similarly, studies suggest that a constant flow of catecholamines may forge neurological pathways that lead a person to be consistently angry and more aggressive all the time. This is directly connected to stress because you only get angry when you're under pressure of some kind. If you don't know how to cope with that pressure, one escape mechanism is blowing up.

As already discussed, individuals under constant stress have trouble processing their emotions. Instead of accepting responsibility for their problems, they may redirect the blame to an outside party and simultaneously become angry and resentful because they know, internally, who is really the guilty party. This constant flow of inner and outer rage leads to the explosive outbursts that some people have—all the result of not knowing how to cope with stress in a healthy way.

Drug, Alcohol, and Tobacco Use

I've now firmly established that if you don't have clear coping mechanisms for dealing with stress, stress will not only affect your life but also your physical, mental, and emotional states. At least on a peripheral level, individuals have a tendency to acknowledge this truth, and they may seek ways to deal with stress…but not necessarily in positive ways. Let's face it—learning new communication skills, going through therapy, addressing past abuse that might have led to one's current reaction to stress, etc., are not easy things to deal with. It's much easier to reach for a supposed quick-fix.

Enter drug, alcohol, and tobacco use. Someone under constant stress desperately wants to find a way to numb the pain. Alcohol, a depressant, (meaning it slows the brain and ANS processes) temporarily serves that function. It makes a person feel like some of the stress has been relieved. In truth, however, the opposite is happening because alcohol actually causes *more* cortisol to be released. It also interferes with how the body processes the glucose that cortisol regulates, and has an impact on insulin sensitivity, which can, over time, lead to diabetes. So, even though a few drinks may seem to ease the sting of a really bad day, inside your body, the alcohol is only making things worse.

For the same reason that individuals under severe stress choose to reach for alcohol, they may also decide to smoke a cigarette (or ten). As with alcohol, cigarettes temporarily seem to lower stress levels. Nicotine triggers the release of dopamine, a "feel good" chemical, in the brain. But…wait for it…nicotine also causes the adrenal glands to release, you guessed it, cortisol. This spikes the heart rate, makes you shake, and does all the things you expect from the fight or flight syndrome. Therefore, smoking actually adds to stress, not relieve it. A study in the *American Psychology Journal* found evidence that adult smokers actually report higher levels of stress than nonsmokers (Parrott, 1999).

Finally, people under duress may reach for a quick remedy in the guise of drugs. Al'Absi Mustafa's research study, "Stress and Addiction: Biological and Psychological Mechanisms," found evidence that individuals who are chronically stressed during childhood, are much more prone to substance abuse due to the chemical damage stress wrought on their neural pathways. Regardless of the drug— marijuana, cocaine, methamphetamines, etc.— temporarily relief, as with alcohol and tobacco, is followed by a rush of cortisol. Consider a cocaine "high," for instance. That's entirely a stress response by the body. Cocaine users feel the same muscular tension, racing heart, dry mouth, and increased strength, that someone in an emergency does.

Thus, based on the many research studies on what these substances do to brain chemistry and the way it mirrors a biological stress response, alcohol, tobacco, and drugs can all definitely be categorized as stress inducers, rather than stress relievers.

Social Withdrawal

By now, you've figured out that stress always comes back to brain chemistry. Social withdrawal is no different. While it may be tempting, when going through a difficult time, to isolate yourself from people to try and "give yourself a break," what actually happens inside your body is counterintuitive. Just as the stress fight or flight response is an evolutionary mechanism, so is a human being's tendency to be a social being. In the Stone Age, there was literally safety in numbers. Our brains developed in such a way that they find social settings comforting, because they were once considered key to survival.

Thus, because our brains literally are wired for social interaction, social withdrawal causes the release of stress hormones. Isolation actually makes you feel worse than if you engaged with others. It becomes a self-perpetuating cycle—you're stressed, so you isolate yourself, so you feel more stressed. Loneliness and social withdrawal lead to disrupted sleep patterns, a weakened immune system, and a decline in cognitive function, all because of the havoc wrought on the brain's chemistry when it is constantly flooded by stress hormones mistakenly trying to defend it from a perceived danger.

Unhealthy Physical Habits

When all else fails to relieve a person's stress, he or she may resort to unhealthy physical habits. Nail biting is one example of a fairly harmless bad habit which some people find self-soothing. Other people crack their knuckles, which is also harmless. But the need for relief from the rush of cortisol and adrenaline also leads people to pull their hair out (trichotillomania), eat nonfood substances (pica), and pick at their skin until they bleed (dermatillomania), among other unhealthy physical habits. Harming your body only stresses it further, so none of this helps an individual trying to find relief.

In the end, you can see that everything relates back to brain chemistry. Man is genetically hardwired for survival, and the brain continues to try to protect him in the twenty-first century the same way it did many millennia ago. However, nowadays, stressors are much less likely to be life-threatening, so it is incumbent upon humans to retrain in their brains how to react appropriately to the daily stresses of modern life. This includes learning ways to cope that don't worsen the situation by further disrupting neural pathways with powerful stress hormones. The first step to finding real stress relief is to know *why* you are stressed. In the next chapter, I'll examine how to recognize when you're stressed (it sounds obvious, but isn't always), what your stress triggers are, and how to become mindfully and emotionally aware.

2

Awareness

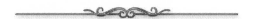

"What is necessary to change a person is to change his awareness of himself."
– Abraham Maslow

When you're stressed, you know you're stressed. Right? I mean, it's obvious when you're under the gun, feeling the effects of cortisol and adrenaline blasting away. Well, maybe not so much. Consider: when you are constantly exposed to anything—music, food, scents, etc.—you eventually develop some sort of tolerance. That's an evolutionary mechanism. In order for human beings to survive, the body developed internal mechanisms to desensitize itself to substances with which it was constantly coming in contact. A modern example of how science applies this to health care is person who is allergic to something. One way to try to help overcome that allergy is immunotherapy, which is literally injecting tiny bits of allergens into the body to gradually desensitize it. How does this relate to stress?

If you're constantly stressed, you sometimes stop realizing you're stressed, because you adapt to always feeling tired, irritated, tense, nervous, etc. You have to adapt, because otherwise you couldn't function on a daily basis, and it starts to just feel normal. Thus, learning how to identify when you're stressed is important to managing it.

We don't always want to admit that we're stressed. We'd rather pretend like we have everything under control instead of asking for help. You have to make sure that you have accepted the fact that your stress is causing bad things to happen in your life before you can take the right steps toward recovery.

RECOGNIZING WHEN YOU ARE STRESSED

Sometimes it's helpful to go down a checklist to try to figure out if something applies to you. While stress responses vary by individual, some general symptoms are common enough that if you notice you have them, you may become stressed out about it. The following symptoms are divided into physical, emotional and behavioral.

Stressful Symptoms

Physical

What does stress feel like? Start with the physical feelings. If you're stressed, you may feel so exhausted that you can barely get out of bed in the morning. Or, conversely, you may feel really wired (as though you've had too much caffeine and are feeling tense and shaky, for instance.) Your head may ache, along with your jaw, neck, shoulders, chest, and back. You may have earaches because of your tense jaw. You may also have stomach cramps and/or digestive difficulties. Your hands might shake or feel cold and clammy. You might not feel any kind of sexual desire at all anymore. One or two of these might just mean you coming down with a cold, but if you're feeling many of these physical symptoms all at once, there's a good chance you're stressed.

Emotional

Next, look at your emotional symptoms. Are you so moody that anything makes you angry? Or so sensitive that you cry for no reason? Do little things that never used to bother you now feel like they completely ruin your day? Does your mind race constantly, such that you can't focus on one single task? Do everyday responsibilities feel like they're weighing you down, overwhelming you to the point where you don't know where to even begin to approach them? Is the glass always half-empty lately? Are you disorganized? Is worry a constant part of your life, even about small, unimportant things? If you're feeling many of these symptoms in tandem, in conjunction with some of the physical symptoms described in the previous paragraph, you are likely to be stressed.

Behavioral

Finally, are you seeing behavioral changes in yourself? Are your eating habits changing (either forgetting to eat meals or suddenly binging, for example)? Are you drinking or smoking more than usual? Are you using drugs when you never did before? Are you biting your nails, picking at your skin, tugging at your hair? Do you pace constantly because sitting feels impossible? Are your organizational habits different (maybe you used to have everything in order on your desk and now it's in total chaos)? Are you procrastinating? All these changes may be signs of stress.

Identifying Triggers

Now you have a good idea of how to recognize when you're stressed. Next, it's important to consider what is causing it. It's helpful to hone in on key triggers because it helps things to feel less overwhelming. When your brain thinks the whole world is attacking it, it's in constant stress mode; and you, understandably, feel that you can't cope. But if you notice that your triggers are specific, you can take action to avoid or address them.

The Mayo Clinic divides stress triggers into major life changes, environment, unpredictable events, workplace and social.

Major Life Changes

Major life changes include death, divorce, moving, a promotion, pregnancy, and family members moving through life stages such as entering school for the first time, leaving for college, or entering a nursing home. All of these, however positive they may sometimes be, can be extremely stressful.

Environment

You are directly impacted by the world around you. If you're walking down the street and a jackhammer suddenly fires up, the loud noise may scare you, make you jump, and trigger a stress response. Loud noises, bright lights, intense heat or cold, animals lunging or barking, and large crowds are all common environmental stressors.

Unpredictable events

Parents dropping by your house unexpectedly, a kid getting sick or getting fired, you name it. If something directly impact the regular routine of your daily life, such an unpredictable event can worry you enough to trigger a full-on stress response.

Workplace

You're at work all day, most days. As such, you're surrounded by what come to feel like normal stressors—

deadlines, demands from your boss, fights with coworkers, wrangling for office supplies, even wondering where to eat lunch, or you don't feel welcome in your office. All these can cause stress. Maybe it's minor stress, initially, but when you're subjected to it, day in and day out, it quickly becomes chronic.

Social

As important as relationships are to our mental and emotional health, they can also be detrimental. Fights with a loved one, worries about dating, arguments with your children, trying to make friends in a new city—people can be as stressful as loneliness.

Make a list of all the things that trigger you. You might not even realize you have any triggers until you sit down and start to think of them. Work your way through each of the categories listed above and pick a few things that consistently trigger a stress response. The key is to find the ones most common to your daily life, not the ones that only rarely ever happen. So focus more on workplace and relationships, for instance, than on unpredictable events. If you discover that a big trigger for you is a particular coworker, for example, then sit down and determine why that coworker bothers you so much. Figure out a way to eliminate that constant stressor, perhaps by addressing the problem, having your desk moved or simply by retraining yourself to look at the situation in a more positive, perhaps humorous light. Once you become aware of your triggers, you will be able to overcome them much easier by either confronting or avoiding them.

There are many different types of stress a person can experience. There are common types that everyone can relate to, but the actual things that stress them out will be different within a category. You might just have one type of stress that you need to overcome, but you might also have an issue with stress in every part of your life. In this section, I'm going to go over the various types of stress you might experience, so you can identify the categories and work through them on an individual level.

Reactions to stress are often different from person to person. Some people internalize their stress, causing depression and a sense of loneliness. Others will externalize their stress, making them angry and irritable. It is important to determine what kind of person you are and how you might handle stress, so you can look for instances of expression within your own life.

You might have more than one kind of stress, leading to a feeling of being overwhelmed. When everything in your life is stressing you out, your body never gets a break! Some people will just have work stress, so they might shut down when they get home, only to get stressed again as they are on their way to work. Others will carry their different types of stress around with them, letting it affect every aspect of their lives. Determine what the root cause of your stress is, so you can better identify the different kinds that you are experiencing.

Workplace Stress

As noted earlier, workplace stress is the norm for most. Day in and day out, everyone feels it in a variety of ways. Since workplace stress is so common, the question becomes, how do know you when it's normal, and how do you know when it has crossed the line into something that is making you sick?

The key, again, is consistency. Look at your daily routine. You undoubtedly have normal stressors like deadlines, a full inbox, coworkers you may butt heads with, a boss who doesn't always seem reasonable, demanding customers, maybe an uncomfortable workspace, hours that are too early or too late, a salary that seems unfair, possibly a long commute to and fro, etc. If you consistently handle these daily stresses without playing them over and over on repeat in your brain, they're probably normal and manageable. Work isn't always fun. This you know for a fact. If the stressors are mere annoyances that you can quickly deal with and set aside, they're not a cause for worry. However, if you're constantly thinking about how much you hate the location, the people, the work, the hours, etc., then you're moving into more dangerous stress territory. If you come home and constantly rant for hours about how awful your day was, can't sleep at night because you're replaying workplace drama in your head, or dread getting out of bed every day, you're very likely stressed in an unhealthy way.

Relationship Stress

The most stressful relationships, by far, are romantic in nature. Romantic relationship stressors start when you begin dating. "Will she like me?" progresses into "Will she *still* like me?" (after you've been dating a while). There's a definite tension involved in keeping romance alive. whether it's new or old. Keeping up appearances can be a stressor—you want to look good for your partner, but you're juggling so many other things and nice clothes/hair/good gym habits, etc., may be difficult to maintain. There's also stress in the bedroom, related to sexual performance. Then there's balancing your work and family life. Or maybe your friends and family don't like your partner. That's yet another stressor. As a relationship evolves, so does the level of stress in it. Even when you eventually come to some kind of comfort level, stress is a normal part of romantic relationships.

Beyond romance, think about the other various tiers of relationships in your life. Start at home. You have your parents. Maybe you also have kids. Next, consider your friends. Finally, factor in people you socialize with outside of family life, such as at work.

All of these relationships, regardless of how close, have a direct impact on your stress level. Such stress isn't all that different from that in a romantic relationship, really, because all relationships require two key things: time and commitment.

Your parents need you to call them occasionally to say hi, but there are only so many hours in the day. Your friends had plans one day to see you outside of work, but you had to drive your kids to sports events and go to your spouse's work awards ceremony, and your parents dropped by unexpectedly... Even your coworkers sometimes require time and energy you don't have. If they ask for help with a project and you turn them down, for instance, it may foster workplace tension.

All of these stressors are normal to everyday life. They only become a problem when they overwhelm you to the point where you're chronically stressed, rather than just shrugging off the usual chaotic day-to-day.

Chronic Stress

Stress can sometimes be just a behavior trait. It might be the way you react and handle particular situations. Some people have trouble pinpointing their sources of stress, feeling as though every little thing stresses them out. This is usually from prolonged exposure to stress, a childhood filled with anxiety, or a traumatic event that hasn't yet been overcome.

Chronic stress usually develops in childhood, when we learned how to use stress as a part of our daily lives. Our parents might have had normalized stress, or it might have become an emotion so familiar that it was all we knew. Some people might be comfortable with stress in their adult lives, even feeling more out of whack when they don't have something to worry over. This is very common and can be difficult to recognize because of its regularity. When our brains developed to be stressed as kids, this condition does not go away easy once we become adults.

Having large secrets can also be a cause of a high level of stress. Individuals who commit a crime without getting caught usually undergo long periods of stress due to the constant fear and worry that they might. Those who have lies might constantly feel stressed or worried as well. People committing adultery, hiding a different personality, or who just want to break up with a partner constantly live under a lot of stress because they don't have the ability to be honest with those around them or themselves.

Chronic stress is, quite bluntly, life-threatening. It affects every organ of your body. It raises blood pressure, can cause breathing problems and digestive issues, impacts the musculoskeletal system, and has a particularly devastating effect on the circulatory system. Ongoing studies suggest that chronic stress may be linked to certain kinds of cancer. All in all, it's vital for your mental, emotional, and physical well-being to learn how to identify and prevent chronic stress.

Positive Stress

Not all stress is harmful. As mentioned, major life events can be stressors, but that doesn't mean they're negative. For example, pregnancy is a huge stress, but it's very often a joyful experience. Moving can be stressful, but it may be offset if due to a promotion or because the new city has exciting opportunities not found in your previous area. Job promotions are stressful because you have brand-new responsibilities, but these also come with a larger salary. Getting married can be very stressful, not just the wedding itself, but learning to coexist with another person every single day. Yet, it can also be the beginning of a wonderful life partnership that offset negative stressors.

Positive stress can challenge you to grow as a person. It helps expand your personal horizons. All in all, the benefits of stress triggers make them well worth the effects they still cause.

MINDFULNESS

Being mindful is one of the easiest ways to overcome stress. It is a practice that takes time to get used to, but once mastered, you will no longer have the overwhelming sensation that comes with stress. Being mindful keeps you away from your constant thoughts; instead, it helps to make sure that you focus on what is important in the current moment. It is not a practice that stops you from being stressed altogether or some sort of hypnosis that makes you a different person. It is just a way to manage stress, anxiety and depression.

It is essentially the attempt to ground an individual in the present instead of the continued rumination of the past and worry over the future. Mindfulness involves becoming aware of one's surroundings and focusing on the present. The more you implement this method into your life, the more you will realize just how disconnected you have been. When you are able to place yourself in the *now* and remove all thoughts away from *then,* you will free your mind from stress and turn those worries into positive inspirations.

Mindfulness is a practice you must do to continually in order to overcome your stress triggers. The more you practice, the better you will get. It is going to be challenging at first, and you might only be able to be mindful for a minute or less while you adjust to this new mindset. That is completely fine, and just remember to continue to practice. The more you do, the better you will address your stress and worries. It is like anything else that takes time. Imagine riding a bike. At first, you might fall off right away. Then you ride for a minute at a time, then five minutes, then ten. Working on improving your mental health takes time, and you have to be willing to practice.

Five Senses

One good method for practicing mindfulness is to make identifications using all five of your senses. You can practice this exercise anytime, anywhere, and it will help you become more aware of your surroundings, helping you focus on something other than stressors and redirecting your racing thoughts to a more positive, grounded mindset.

Find something to smell. You don't have to get up and retrieve the item. Instead, look around the room and identify something you could smell at any given moment. Maybe you are in the kitchen and see a salt shaker sitting on the counter. Perhaps you are at work and there is an office plant sitting on your coworker's desk. Point this thing out as a way to ground yourself in the moment.

Search for something to taste. Again, you don't want to actually get up and get that item. Instead, you want to identify the object. Think of a pepper shaker, for instance, imagine what a few grains of pepper would taste like on your tongue, and identify the factors of taste surrounding the chosen object.

Identify something you see. This is the easiest one to do. Just look at the thing in front of you and see it. Don't think too deeply about any of these commands during the stages. They should be done within a couple of seconds. If you stop and take a moment too long for each item, you will likely find that you begin to ruminate or worrying once again. Instead, move through the activity as quickly as possible.

Pick out something you hear. Is there a dog barking outside, or can you hear the clock ticking that is hanging on the wall? Maybe the person you are sitting with is tapping his feet, or perhaps you are moving your own. If the room is completely silent, what do you hear? Is there a guitar sitting in the corner? Is there a large box that you could throw across the room to make a loud sound if you really wanted to?

Discover something you can touch. This should an item so close that you can actually touch it. This is one of the stages where you would want to run your fingers over an object. Maybe it is a pair of velvet pants or perhaps the fur of the cat sitting next to you. When you can touch something and associate your sense to your thoughts, you finally ground yourself in the moment and become completely aware of only the present.

You should do this activity within a couple of minutes in your mind. Afterward, you will hopefully have moved on from whatever stressful thoughts you were allowing to run through your head. If not, repeat the activity with different identifying factors. Maybe think of a specific category, such as things that are green or that start with a certain letter of the alphabet. By doing this, you will focus attention on your current state rather than where you have been or where you are going.

Group Mindfulness

Playing games is a great way to make a group mindful. These don't always have to be competitive games but, instead, something you can all work on together, such as a puzzle.

Eating dinner at the table is better than doing it in front of the TV. Instead of focusing on the people you are watching, the people you are sharing a meal with will instead help you focus on the present moment, discussing lives, interacting and connecting.

In a business setting, you can strive for group interaction. Have continual meetings with one another to ensure that you are staying connected with coworkers. The more you can be mindful in a moment, the better off you will all be.

Meditation

Meditation is another great tool for someone who wants to practice mindfulness. It is much harder to practice for beginners trying to overcome their stress. Before you start, make sure that you fully understand what it takes to be mindful, so that take the proper steps needed to find peace within yourself.

Start the process of meditation by finding a location you can dedicate to this practice. If you try to meditate in the same spot where you do other things, it might be harder for your brain to fully shut down and relax. For example, instead of sitting on your bed, you might want to sit next to it by your end table, in a place you wouldn't normally sit. Once you start to associate this location with relaxing, your mind will be able to easily zone out and focus on finding peace rather than going through the usual stressful thoughts.

To meditate, begin by letting go of your thoughts. Yes, your mind is undoubtedly full with the events of the day, the chores you haven't done yet, the little annoyances on constant replay at the back of your brain. Accept that they are there, and then switch your focus to your breathing. Imagine that your mind is a river and thoughts are boats. Just let them float downstream, paying no attention to them. Instead, focus on a slow and steady inhale and exhale.

Don't judge yourself if you struggle to focus on something besides your busy mind. It's okay. With practice, you'll be able to send those ships down the river and move into a restful state where your brain can take a break from the daily chaos.

If you're new to meditation, start with five minutes of sitting quietly, focusing on your breath. You can extend the time later, if you'd like. But at the outset, just give yourself those five minutes to reset your brain. That's what meditation does. Science has proved that regular meditation literally rewires the brain in an exceedingly positive way. Research shows that regular meditation may very well lessen the likelihood of cognitive decline and diseases such as Alzheimer's.

No matter how busy you might be, everyone has five minutes a day during which they can focus on different forms of meditation and breathing exercises. The benefits are well worth investing the small bit of time and effort it takes to make this a daily habit.

Emotional Intelligence

Emotional intelligence is the ability to measure your own emotions as well as other people's. When you understand why you might be feeling a certain way as well as why others around you might have certain thoughts or emotions, you can better regulate your feelings and avoid anything negative that might come along with the inability to control how you feel.

Those with a high level of emotional intelligence usually have a higher level of intelligence and awareness, making it easier to identify different feelings. If you are a very emotionally aware person, you can easily pinpoint why you might be feeling a certain way as well as why others might be behaving in a certain manner. When you do this, you can identify your own triggers and improve your own mood which, in turn, will help people around you, who may be dealing with their own stressors.

Now that you've learned to identify when you're stressed, what specific kind of stress you might be feeling, and what could have triggered that stress, you're better equipped to learn how to effectively manage it. The coping strategies shared in this chapter, such as meditation, are the start to a whole new healthy way of handling stress. That said, what if you could prevent stress? Then you wouldn't have to cope with it in the first place. There will always be stress, of course. But if you can learn to prevent at least some of it, you'll feel that much less overwhelmed. Forewarned is forearmed!

3

Prevention

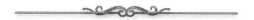

"An ounce of prevention is worth
a pound of cure."
– Benjamin Franklin

As discussed in the previous chapter, one of the first steps in coping with stress is identifying the stressor and then the specific kind of stress experienced. After you know what is causing your body to produce stress hormones, you can consider how to prevent it from happening. Naturally, there are situations where you have no control. An unreasonably demanding boss, for instance, isn't something you can change, unless you switch jobs. An hour-long commute may be unavoidable on a daily basis, no matter how early you get up. And there may be relationships in your life you can't avoid but that cause a great deal of tension. So what do you do in these situations?

The key is to have a game plan for when stressful situations arise, whether anticipated or not. It's possible you have plans for other parts of your life such as what to do in the event of a hurricane or fire. These are ways of ensuring that someone knows what to do in a crisis. It gives you a method to the madness, if you will, as you methodically work your way through each step of your disaster plan.

In this chapter, creating goals to manage stress will be discussed. Setting goals helps you identify clear targets. In a fire escape plan, you identify doors to evacuate through. With a stress goal plan, you begin the process of identifying a different kind of door—a stress relief exit.

Then we will discuss techniques for avoiding stressful situations. Of course, they can't all be avoided, but if you have a good grasp of basic techniques, you'd be surprised how much your stress can be side-stepped.

Finally, I will teach you a mindset to help create as stress-free an environment as possible. Since the world is already a stressful place, knowing how to mentally minimize stress in the places where you spend most of your time is incredibly helpful.

CREATING GOALS

Most people suffer stress in more than one area of their lives. As such, you can potentially set one goal for each major area—but not all at once! People's lives can broadly be divided into the following categories:

- **Relationships**
- **Work (or education, for those in school)**
- **Finances**
- **Health**

Each of these areas, of course, can also be subdivided.

In the following section I will briefly work through each major area. However, it bears repeating—you should *not* set a goal for every single area. Not yet, anyway.

Relationships

Your immediate family, your significant other, friends, acquaintances, coworkers, or classmates—these are all some of the types of relationships you probably participate in on a near-daily basis. And each one of them has the possibility of creating its own unique stressor. Sometimes, you can end up stressed by multiple relationship conflicts. Perhaps more than any other stressor, relationships can really push you to the breaking point. How do you use goals to help you cope?

Ever hear of the story of the blind men and the elephant? A group of blind men were placed before an elephant. Since they were blind, they had to touch the unfamiliar animal in order to assess it. One man felt the trunk and decided the elephant was a snake. The man who touched just the tail insisted it was a rope. And on and on. They built their perceptions based specifically on the part of the elephant they were examining. What does any of this have to do with goal setting?

Goals are uniquely helpful in that they require you to zero in on a target, putting metaphorical blinders on as you strive to reach a particular aim. Sometimes you need blinders in relationships to help you focus on just one area of conflict. While that might very well spider-web into other relationships, focusing initially on "one piece of elephant [read: relationship] at a time" is a start.

Work or Education

Whether you're in an office all day or a classroom, or any other work or educational setting, you're bombarded by stressors on any number of levels. (Stressors beyond work/school relationships were addressed in the previous section.) Everything from deadlines and malfunctioning software to money to pay for textbooks to an uncomfortable workspace or wondering about a long-overdue promotion is a stressor.

We spend so much of our lives in work or school. It's only natural that in survey after survey, these two areas are considered the biggest stressors in a person's life, after relationships. One of the reasons they're so stressful is that there are so many parts. The commute to work (or school), your personal work area, the many tasks you're required to complete on a daily basis, your salary (or tuition)—stress can arise due to any or all of those. Again, you want to zero in on one area with your goal and address it first, rather than tackling the whole elephant at once.

Say your workspace is physically uncomfortable. Well, why? Is it the temperature? Your chair? The lighting? Choose what's most critical to your comfort on a daily basis and then set a goal to take appropriate action, whether that's talking to Human Resources about a more ergonomic setup or leaving a sweater at work, so it's always there if a coworker cranks down the thermostat.

Finances

Money. The root of all evil? Who knows? But definitely a major stressor in all our lives. Consider this rather absurd but true story: a woman spent a good part of her life worrying about not making enough money. Then she opened her own company and started earning a good salary for the first time. She even made enough to start building a nice nest egg. Wonderful, right? Well, tax season rolled around and, because she was self-employed, had few deductibles, and had earned a decent amount of money, her tax bill wiped out all the savings of the last year. The tax accountant informed her that most self-employed businesses don't make it past the second year because the tax bill is more than what the business is earning. Ouch.

We worry about earning little money. We worry about earning too much. We worry about what do with the money we have—where to put it, who to share it with, what to buy or not. If we have children, we worry about teaching them to be financially re-sponsible. All in all, money, as necessary as it is to our lives, is a constant stressor. That's why setting finan-cial goals can be so helpful.

While you may have any number of financial problems, such as a variety of debts or monthly bills, choosing a goal to pay down one by a specific date is a way to help you feel less overwhelmed. One debt at a time. When it's cleared, move on to the next issue, such as whether or not to invest. Etc.

Health

Stress can affect your health. And health can affect your stress. Can it ever! Things may be going just fine in all other areas of your life, but even a simple cold can cause stress to feel like it's lurking around every corner. You're tired. You're achy. Every small problem suddenly becomes magnified. And that's just a common cold. If you're dealing with a chronic, debilitating illness, your stress levels are undoubtedly (and understandably) high. Beyond the financial impact of having to pay for insurance, doctor's copays, etc., you're dealing with the emotional stress of either you or a loved one not feeling well. You're coping with sudden limitations to what you can physically and mentally do.

Health is unique in that it's much harder to use the "elephant" approach to goal-set. Once you're ill, you're ill, and you have to somehow deal with all the ramifications. So a good goal could very well be to avoid additional illnesses (or mitigate existing ones) by adopting self-health practices such as exercise or meditation. It's important to remember that your physical, mental, and emotional well-being are all tied together. One affects the other like a chain of falling dominos. Therefore, this is one area where establishing a truly focused goal can be of great use. For example, taking time to meditate ten minutes a day has been scientifically proven to benefit all areas of health.

The above are all areas where you can set goals. Bear in mind what has been said earlier, —don't set more than one goal initially. Remember that goal-setting in and of itself can be stressful. Putting aside other goals and focusing on just one can trigger stress hormones. Setting a specific date to achieve something and not succeeding can be very stressful. Be realistic and kind to yourself when goal setting. Follow these steps:

1. Take one of the areas listed above and brainstorm a list of stresses.

2. Cull that list down to one stressor that you want to address at the present moment.

3. Verbalize your goal so that it's reasonable *and* measurable. For instance, "By May 15, I will have gotten a doctor's note to share with Human Resources about needing an ergonomic desk to help with my carpal tunnel syndrome." Notice that you're not immediately saying, "I will have a brand-new desk by May 15." You're taking the first step toward getting that desk by obtaining an important note.

4. Write the goal on a sticky note and post it on the mirror where you get dressed in the morning. While it may sound ridiculous, saying it out loud each day whelps you remember what you're planning to achieve and by when.

5. Not all goals require multiple steps, but if they do, make sure you take the elephant apart, piece by piece. Maybe your first goal is to get the note. Then your next goal is to talk to HR. And your final goal is to have that chair in

place by June 1. Be methodical in your approach to achieving your desired result.

6. After you have accomplished your goal, reward yourself! You did something great to begin lowering your stress.

7. Repeat these steps for your next goal.

All this undoubtedly sounds like it may take a very long time. And yes, it can. Eventually, you'll start setting multiple goals at once. But while you're learning the process, stick to one to avoid adding counterintuitive stress to what should be a destressing practice.

These are possible goals you might set, based on your personal needs:

- I will buy a pedometer and make sure I walk 5,000 steps a day this month.
- I will meditate for five minutes three times a week.
- I will meet with my financial advisor on x date and discuss a specific target for my savings account.
- I will sit down with [relationship] and calmly discuss x problem, which we've been avoiding forever.

TECHNIQUES FOR AVOIDING
STRESSFUL SITUATIONS

One of the biggest problems with stress is that sometimes it feels unavoidable to the point of being suffocating. You look around and see problems everywhere. You don't know how to begin to tackle so many conflicts, and a dark cloud of stress descends on you and everything feels heavy and painfully difficult to slog through, with no end in sight. While you can't circumvent every obstacle, there are things you can do to avoid stressful situations as much as possible.

Learn to Manage Your Time

One stress you can avoid is the deadly late-for-work/school-or-a-deadline rush. It's all a manner of organizing and prioritizing. Commit to spending a little bit of time each Sunday listing your most critical, time-sensitive tasks for the coming week. List them in order of priority. Identify which you need to perform and which you can have other people do. Then mark them on a calendar with some kind of very simple code like red for "URGENT." (This is stressful, but it serves a purpose.) Commit to checking one task off that calendar every single day.

If one of your stressors is always being late, lay your clothes out the night before. Consider showering at night. Put your alarm clock across the room so you have to get up to turn it off—and then don't go back to bed! Make your breakfast ahead of time (and lunch, maybe!)

Just doing these two things can make a world of difference in your stress level.

Learn to Delegate

This goes back to the list you made on Sunday. Learn to share your workload, whether it's by assigning chores to children or your significant other, or by delegating at the office. This isn't always possible, but more often than not, we take on way more than we should. People are always willing to help.

That said, yes, it's stressful to turn important work over to someone else. If you do, you know it'll be done right. So this particular technique requires committing to learning to trust a little bit. No, the work may not turn out exactly to your standard. Learn to accept that, so long as it's still good quality. Everything doesn't *have* to be five-star. Pick the tasks that should be done by you, and let other people handle tasks of a less vital nature. And if you get to work and the report isn't formatted quite the way you want it or you come home and your kid only half vacuumed the living room... it's okay. Acceptance is a big part of managing stress. Delegate when possible. Then accept the results (within reason). It requires letting go of some control. And that automatically removes weight from your shoulders, even if initially it feels dangerous.

Prioritize Time for Yourself

As busy as you are, you're no good to yourself or anyone else if you're a stressed-out wreck. Set a time on your calendar where, each day, you do something good for your mental health. As much as possible, do not skip that personal appointment. It doesn't have to be fancy. It could be taking five minutes to have your morning coffee on the porch, enjoying the new day. It could be a fifteen-minute walk every day. Or taking the stairs instead of the elevator—unhurriedly—more as mental than physical exercise. You could commit to starting to meditate just a few minutes a day. Just ten minutes a day of some "you" activity will do wonders for your physical, mental, and emotional health and, by default, for your stress level.

Find a Support System

Life is too hard to go it alone. One of the best things you can do to avoid stress is to find a good, consistent support system. Sometimes it's easier said than done, but it doesn't have to be hard. A support system can be as simple as meeting a dear friend once a week for a cup of coffee, without fail. Knowing you'll be able to touch base with her and tell her all about the highs and lows of the week will be something to look forward to.

If you're going through a particular kind of stress, such as a health crisis (you or someone else) or divorce, look up support groups online. There exist for everything from cancer support groups to mental health communities. Most major groups have ways to call, email or chat, and they may help you find a regular support person you can contact on a daily basis. The key is to reach out. These groups exist. All you have to do is Google "online support groups" and a huge variety will pop up for almost any crisis you may be enduring. You are *not* alone. You can also ask your doctor to refer you to a therapist, if your stress is affecting you on a mental and emotional level. Or seek a referral from a trusted friend.

Once you find one of these groups or get a referral, make sure you follow up and continue to do so. The only way your support system will truly help you is if you're consistent in asking for the help you need.

CREATING A STRESS-FREE ENVIRONMENT

Let's be clear. In this section, I'm not talking about a stress-free physical location. Some of these exist, yes, but not many. The goal here is to discuss steps you can take to help your mind feel less stress. Your brain is what produces stress hormones that then run rampant and lead to fight-or-flight chaos. If you can do specific things to help calm your mind, your environment will naturally feel that much less stressful. Granted, sometimes you may have to change physical locations in order to help your amygdalae relax. It all depends on your particular needs.

Emphasize Communication

Specific individuals may be stressing you out, or they have the power to help you address another stressor (such as an HR rep who can help you with a coworker you feel uncomfortable around). When discussing it, think of the word *talk* and not *complain*. Take time to reflect on what is stressing you specifically. Identify what *you* personally can and cannot change. Then take steps to communicate the situation. Keeping quiet may feel safe but it's the worst thing you can do for your stress level. The conflict will just continue to bubble and boil inside you until it finally bursts out in some kind of nasty altercation.

Set aside time in a neutral location (where neither of you will feel like you're on the other person's "turf") to talk about the problem. Use "I feel/because" statements rather than "You did this" or "It's your fault." So, "I felt angry when you contradicted me in front of the children today because we didn't present a united front" versus "You make me so mad when you don't agree with me in front of the kids!" Be specific about the situation that upset you.

Then present a possible solution, "It would be helpful to me if, when I discipline Bob at the dining room table, you don't disagree immediately. If you have concerns, please address them with me afterwards, in private, and I'll make sure to listen and consider taking a different approach next time."

You can use this approach with any kind of relationship. "I feel/because," followed by a clear solution. If the person you're talking to doesn't like the solution, that's okay. You may not resolve the conflict immediately. The fact that you are communicating and starting to address an issue—and you continue to communicate until the problem is resolved and thereafter to ensure other problems don't arise—will be a huge factor in creating a stress-free mental environment.

Prioritize Time for Yourself

Wait. Didn't you see this one already in the previous section? Yes. That's because it bears repeating. The more you set aside specific time for your physical, mental, and emotional health, the more stress-free your environment will be. While you may not love exercising, going for a regular walk will help you from head to toe, including your mood and stress level.

Prioritizing time for yourself can involve regularly scheduling a clean-up of your personal space. If you have files all over the place at work, your stress level is going to be high because you'll probably lose things. Seeing so many files will also remind you of how many tasks remain unresolved. So, make keeping your personal space neat, uncluttered, and comfortable a priority.

Schedule regular time to meet with friends or family. This isn't a luxury. It's absolutely vital to your mental health and stress level.

Regular checkups are also a part of prioritizing time for yourself. Don't skip a doctor's appointment because you're overwhelmed with work. You are more important than work. You only have one body and one brain. Once damaged, you can't replace them. Take care of yourself, inside and out.

Remove Yourself from the Situation

Easier said than done, right? But sometimes, it's vital. If your work environment is toxic to the point where you simply can't fix the constant problem, you may want to consider switching jobs. It's a drastic move, absolutely. But remember that chronic stress can and will damage your health. However stressful switching jobs is, developing a chronic health condition is far worse. You don't have to do it overnight. Set a goal. Maybe you want to polish your resume by a certain date. Then set another goal. Maybe you want to start looking for jobs and apply to x number by x date. And then maybe you want to take a couple days off to go interview. Etc. Be methodical, using the tools you learned earlier.

Similarly, if you're living way too far from places you need to be every day, and the stress of coming and going is becoming impossible to bear, it's worth looking for a new home, even if it may be a slow process. Take it slow and steady. Don't rush into it and make things even harder on yourself. Also, don't stay in a situation where your health is going to ultimately suffer on all levels.

Or it could be that your house is just fine, but the people in that house are making things unbearable. If communication and therapy don't help at all, it may be time to look at alternative living arrangements.

Whatever your particular situation, there's always a way to minimize stress. It just requires taking time to honestly reflect on what the problem is. Then, following the steps outlined in this chapter, set reasonable, measurable goals. Some of these goals might be practicing the stress-relieving techniques provided. For example, you might decide to set a stress-relieving time-management goal such as, "I will schedule thirty minutes every Sunday for one month to plan out my activities for the following week." Finally, take into account the impact of a stress-free mental environment and take steps to ease the pressure on your overactive, stress-hormone-producing amygdalae.

In the next chapter, I'll address the everyday activities that lower stress, including suggested exercises for both mental and physical stress relief. All of these activities require a small time commitment, so you'll need to use time-management strategies to avoid further stress. But that time commitment is vital to your well-being and to the overall goal of this book—

teaching you how to find stress relief in concrete, practical ways that are applicable to your daily life.

4

Action

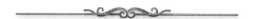

"An idea not coupled with action will never get
any bigger than the brain cell it occupied."
– Arnold Glasow

Once you have become aware of what stress is, how it is caused, and how it is prevented, you now have the tools to take action and confront the stress that lives in your life, either addressing and mitigating it, or outright eliminating it. In previous chapters, I've discussed techniques you can apply. Now I'll go a step further and discuss everyday activities that can, with consistent practice, help lower stress.

Science has proven again and again that exercise is a huge part of combating stress. As such, in this chapter I'll discuss simple exercises you can incorporate into your daily life that will help you relieve stress and induce relaxation. Given the fact that everyone has differing amounts of free time, exercises will be categorized as one-minute, five-minute, etc., so you can choose the routine that best suits your lifestyle. Additionally, I've categorized the various exercises by specific goals. For example, if you want to sleep better, go straight to that exercise.

This will help you establish a plan to deal with chronic stress and provide you with the tools to consistently follow up by checking in on yourself on a weekly, monthly, and yearly basis. Depending on your stress level, you'll have a concrete plan in place to address it.

EVERYDAY ACTIVITIES TO LOWER STRESS

On a daily basis, each and every one already does certain things to help reduce stress. Some activities are conscious. For example, using a stress ball is a common way that individuals reduce stress-related muscular tension. Other activities may not even be noticed, such as comfort eating. Whatever you already are or aren't doing to ease your stress, there are many activities you can incorporate into your daily routine to help you relax.

In this section, I'll review a number of different activities and provide you with a plan so you can add them into your daily life without added stress.

One of the key activities for lowering everyday stress, which costs nothing, is taking a daily walk. Many studies have shown that walking is beneficial on multiple levels. It helps you physically, obviously, but it can also be meditative—and meditation, as noted, has been proven to be an effective stress-fighting tool. If, as you walk, you practice letting go of the negativities of the day and, instead, focus on all the pleasant things around that you're passing by, or make a mental list of some of the good things you may have forgotten happened during the day. Thus, you're incorporating a kind of walking meditation into your lifestyle. But whether you're walking fast or slow, studies are conclusive: adding a daily walk is a proven way to consistently combat stress and also help you prevent further stress by raising your endorphin level.

Exercise

Countless studies done detail the healthy impact exercise has on a person's body from head to toe. The salutatory effects of exercise directly influence the production of stress hormones. As you may recall, stress starts in your amygdala which signals your hypothalamus to radio your body's nervous system. In turn, your nervous system reacts by producing stress hormones such as cortisol and adrenaline.

Various studies at Harvard University found that aerobic exercise lessens one's levels of adrenaline and cortisol. More importantly, moderate exercise triggers the release of endorphins, your body's "feel-good" hormones. So, when you exercise, you're tackling stress on two key levels—you're lowering it. And you're also raising endorphin levels to help prevent it.

Possibilities for exercise include dancing, self-defense classes, bowling, a walk around your neighborhood at a moderate pace, roller blading, Pilates, swimming, yoga, gardening (more physical than you'd think!), and weightlifting. Aim for at least thirty minutes a day of your chosen exercise to maximize the total health benefits—mental, physical, and emotional.

Relaxation

Most people wouldn't necessarily call exercise "relaxing." It helps destress you in different ways than outright relaxation, which is also an effective way to deal with daily stress. You can look at relaxation as "me time." It's time for *you*. No one else. There are enough demands throughout your day. When you commit to incorporating periods of relaxation into your daily schedule, while initially it may be stressful -- such that you think "I can't find time!" -- it's worth that small initial stress. You'll soon find that the benefits of spending a minimum of fifteen minutes relaxing outweigh the little bit of stress you encounter when you have to put aside another pressing chore to focus on yourself instead.

Yes, you may have children. Or a significant other who wants to spend time with you. Friends or relatives who ask to bend your ear. A list of tasks a mile high. And you'll do every one of these things better if you consistently make time for relaxing. That's a promise. You'll be more patient with your children. More positive with anyone you converse with. More efficient as an employee. Try it for a week—you really have to commit, to see the effects—and you'll see the wholesale difference it makes in your mindset.

How do you do it? Make an initial commitment for fifteen minutes a day. Then stick to it. There's no real "best time" for this. Some people find it easiest to get up a little earlier. Others incorporate relaxation into a lunch break, putting aside all work and focusing, instead, solely on easing the foot off the gas pedal. Still others get their relaxation on the commute. The key is consistency.

Possible activities you can try include listening to music (great for a commute), reading a chapter of a book, soaking in the bath, getting a cup of coffee from your favorite café, catching a catnap, watching a movie (even if you only watch it in fifteen-minute increments initially, you'll still find yourself relaxing and anticipating the next TV session), getting a massage, doing a puzzle, painting, or meditating. As long as it's time just for you, with no pressure, deadlines, or demands from others, it's relaxing.

PRACTICAL STRESS-RELIEF EXERCISES

In the previous section, I discussed ways to help you relieve stress on a daily basis. In this section, I'll provide additional exercises that, when consistently incorporated into your daily routine, can help lower your stress hormones.

These exercises take anywhere from one minute to ten minutes. No matter which you choose, you'll feel calmer and more relaxed from head to toe after practicing even one of them.

Try each exercise throughout the course of a week or two. See which ones you like best and can refer back to as needed on a busy day when you need a quick break.

If you have five minutes, you can do all five exercises in a row. Or if you only have three minutes, do three. Use these exercises in whatever way is most helpful to you.

One-Minute Exercises

Below are a few one-minute exercises that will instantly relieve stress. You can do these activities almost anywhere:

1. Choose a part of your body at random. Flex this muscle as hard as you can for one second, releasing instantly. The relief you feel after-

ward can be enough to reduce stress instantly. Don't strain yourself and don't overdo it.

2. Breathe in through your nose while counting to ten. Then swallow once and hold your breath for one second. Purse your lips and expel your breath while counting to ten once more. Do this three times within a minute.

3. Lightly run the fingers of one hand across the palm on the opposite hand, moving up and down each finger. Repeat twice, then do the same with the other hand. This a surprisingly easy, relaxing activity.

4. Close your eyes. For one minute, slowly count the times you inhale and exhale. There aren't any number of "required" breaths. Just breathe in and out, focusing on the sensation of your chest rising and falling. When you open your eyes after the minute has ended, you'll feel much lighter overall.

5. Walk outside and take one minute to stare at the horizon. This is more pleasant if it's a nice view, of course, but even if it's not, focus your eyes on a distant point and then count your breaths for the minute. Don't focus hard— just rest your eyes lightly. Rest. That's the key. If you can do this for two or three minutes, so much the better.

Five-Minute Exercises

When you have a little more time, these are good exercises for you. Try them before going back to work, after a lunch break or when preparing for an important, stressful event:

1. Close your eyes and visualize a place you want to be. Maybe it is wrapped up in warm blankets in your bed. Perhaps you have chosen to visualize a beach. Wherever this happy place is, go there for a moment, feeling everything good that comes along. When you open your eyes, try to mimic those same good feelings, only in the current place you are.

2. Next time you are searching online, if you come across a funny video, save it to your personal files. Keep a collection of videos and pictures that you find amusing. Watch or look at them, making sure you actually laugh out loud. Watching one five-minute video can elicit a feeling of happiness that will stick with you throughout the day.

3. Pick a simple exercise that you can do almost anywhere. A squat, a push-up, a jumping jack, and a sit-up are all exercises that require no equipment. Next time you feel stressed, try one. If all these exercises sound awful, just find a set of stairs and run up and back down.

Just a five-minute exercise can carry you through the rest of the day.

4. Take out a piece of paper and spend five minutes listing positive things that happened in the day. If you can't think of anything good for today, list the positive things in your life. There's always something, whether it's a roof that doesn't leak, clean water to drink, or a safe home to return to at night. At the end of the five minutes, read over the list and realize that, however bad things may sometimes seem, there's a lot of good stuff amid the chaos. You'll be surprised—and relieved.

5. This one is going to sound absurd, but trust me, it works. Go into the bathroom. Set a timer on your phone for three minutes. Then wash your hands. As you're scrubbing away, imagine that you're washing away all the negative stuff that happened today that is stressing you out. After time is up, spend two more minutes drying your hands slowly and methodically with a paper towel. As you're drying, mentally list as many positive things as you can in your life either today or any other day. (See number four, above, for ideas.)

Ten-Minute Exercises

When you have a little more time to spare, these are good exercises to try for stress relief:

1. Ten minutes of meditation is all that is needed in a day. If you are at work and have no place to meditate, try going to your car and sitting quietly just for a few minutes. Even if you have to go to the bathroom, use this quiet and simple space as a location as a place where you can close your eyes and focus on something else.

2. Get a notebook, sketch pad, or open a new Word document. Set a timer for ten minutes. Then write or doodle whatever pops into your head, without stopping. Don't think about what's going down on the paper; just keep writing or drawing until the timer goes off. If you run out of things, draw random lines. The goal is to keep your pen or pencil moving. Afterwards, either tear the page out and throw it away or save it for future reference. You'll feel much better having gotten out some of the stuff that was inside you, even if it doesn't necessarily seem coherent on the page.

3. Give yourself a ten-minute massage. It never feels as good to rub our own back or feet as getting a massage from someone else, but it can still be greatly helpful. Start with your toes, working your way up your legs. Massage your neck and shoulders as best you can, just so you can feel more connected to your body while also relieving pressure.

4. Make yourself a cup of tea or coffee. Don't get it from a vending machine. Set a timer. Then go through the routine of boiling the water and waiting for the tea to steep or for the coffee to percolate. As you're waiting, focus on the activity before you, such as the water dripping down or the steam drifting from the cup. Stay in the present moment. This should take roughly five to seven minutes. When your drink is ready, use the remaining minutes to really savor it, rather than gulping it like you usually do. Even after your time is up, you'll still have some left over to enjoy the moment and relax.

5. Go online and YouTube "Marconi Union – Weightless (Official Video)." Neuroscientists in the UK have found that people who watch this video have sixty-five percent lower stress levels. The video is 8:08 minutes long, so use the last two minutes to close your eyes and count your breaths until time is up. By the end of the ten minutes, you'll feel, well, weightless.

EXERCISES FOR TARGETED GOALS

It is time now to practice methods of combating specific stress. Stress affects everyone differently, so it is important to know how to address an exact issue.

You will notice a reduction in your stress level once you change your lifestyle, but as previously mentioned, human bodies have become used to the stress, so we have to make sure we're retraining different parts as well. These exercises are goal-specific. Look for one that targets a particular stressor, such as feeling agitated, and use it as appropriate to relieve your tension.

Easing Agitation

Many of the activities mentioned in this book are helpful in reducing stress overall. If you are particularly concerned about achieving a level of calmness, another exercise can help. It is another breathing exercise that involves your nose and two fingers.

Pinch your nose as if you were stopping yourself from smelling something bad. Lift your finger off the right nostril and breathe in while counting to four. Hold for one count and place your finger back on your right nostril, lifting your other finger off the left nostril. Breathe out for a count of four. Repeat this with the opposite nostril. You will find that you are instantly calm even after just one time of this breathing exercise.

Stopping Headaches

Headaches are a common stress reaction. Unfortunately, they're also uniquely equipped to derail not just your mood but also your focus. It's impossible to be alert or feel positive when your head is pounding so much that even your eyes ache. You'll know you have a stress headache because it won't just be your forehead. You're feel it in your very muscles, through your jaw, possibly down to your neck.

When you feel that stress headache setting in, consider whether you've had enough to drink. Dehydration exacerbates headaches. While you take whatever medicine you use (maybe the one your doctor prescribed), also drink a few cups of water.

If your headache persists, practice any of the breathing exercises discussed in this book. Focus on your breathing, rather than on your head, and notice the expansion and contraction of your chest, rhythmically inhaling and exhaling for several minutes.

Also try tilting your head from right to left, to the front, and to the back, all while counting to at least ten. You will start to feel the pressure release from your shoulders and neck, eventually relieving your headache as well. It took awhile for the pain to build, so it won't disappear all at once. The level of pain should gradually decrease, however, as you attempt these exercises. Remember, if you catch the headache when it first starts, and do one of the stress-relieving exercises discussed in this book, you'll get relief much faster.

Release Muscle Tension

When stressed, your muscles can easily become tense because human bodies react in a way that prepares us for whatever methods of combat we may need to elicit. When too stressed, we will start to feel sore and achy all over because we have kept our muscles so tense.

Water and sleep will help the most with this, but there are some instant fixes. First off, tell yourself to relax your muscles. Start with your shoulders and jaw. Those usually hold the most tension. Let your jaw hang as naturally as possible. Try to not have a clenched jaw whatsoever. While you do this, let your shoulders drop as well. If you are having trouble with this, try pretending there is a weight that is pulling them down.

Then release the muscles that are working on making things drop downward, and you will reach a happy medium. Alternate between your jaw and your shoulders. When you go back to one, you will realize that you were likely already clenching the other one back up. Repeat this as often as possible all throughout your day. There's no reason or productive benefit of holding so much tension in your shoulders all throughout the day.

Getting Sleep

While sleep is vital to managing stress, sometimes you just can't get your mind to stop racing. You need to do an exercise, while lying in bed, to help you relax and sink into slumber. One such exercise, suggested by the National Sleep Foundation, is doing what has been suggested earlier in this book—focusing on your breathing, noticing the sensation of air entering and exiting your nose, and watching your chest rise and fall. When you've done this for at least two minutes, then do a full-body scan. Starting at the top of your head, imagine that you're directing a laser over your body. Let it move slowly and steadily, lingering only when it finds a tense spot. When this happens, breathe in and out slowly, and imagine that light is filling this place, breaking up the tension. Continue the scan until you get to your toes. At this point, you should start to feel sleepy.

One thing to consider if you're stressed out and struggling to sleep is what scientists call "sleep hygiene." It's important to use your bedroom for relaxing. No work at all while in bed! You want it to be a place that your body and mind associate with total rest. Furthermore—and this one, you won't like, but it's scientifically proven—do not take your electronics to bed with you. No cell phones or laptops. At least thirty minutes before bed, give technology a pass? Why? Because such devices emit a "blue" light that disrupts how your body produces melatonin, a critical sleep hormone. Over and over, studies have shown that blue light disruption sends your body's natural sleep system haywire. So read a book or do something else before bed and you'll soon reap the benefits a good night's rest has on your stress level.

PLANNING TO DEAL WITH CHRONIC STRESS

Chronic stress is what it sounds like—unrelenting stress. Like a chronic disease, stress can literally shift your body from the inside out. Evidence that suggests that nonstop stress can cause cell mutation and lead to cancer. Chronic anything isn't good, let's face it, and chronic stress can be deadly in the long run.

That said, how do you deal with chronic stress? Some stressors there's just no escaping. For example, if you have a critically ill loved one at home, and you're the primary caregiver, that's an unrelenting chronic stressor, no matter how much you care about the person. You can't change the situation, or many others that cause chronic stress, but you can control how you react to it, at least. Two ways to do this are goal setting and personal check-ins. I've discussed goal setting before and it's so important to mention it again here. Personal check-ins, you'll see, just make common sense and are another key way to helping you cope with chronic stress.

Goal Setting

Earlier in this book, I discussed the importance of setting goals to help you cope with stress. I reviewed various areas in your life and suggested ways to target particular problems, sending measurable, reasonable goals to help you ease your stress, a little at a time.

When it comes to overcoming chronic stress, it's important to set a long-term goal for yourself. The stress isn't going anyway. But you can establish parameters wherein you can consistently cope with I in a t healthy way.

For example, you might commit to exercising several times a week. The first goal you set will be to get a gym membership. The next might be to buy gym clothes. Another might be to actually go to the gym, twice a week, for a month. Be methodical in your goal setting. You'll find the payoff well worth the effort.

Check-Ins

Data is all the rage in many industries right now. Education, business, health care... they all emphasize the importance of gathering information that can then be used to track students/employees/patients, etc. When you're dealing with chronic stress, gathering data can be very useful for assessing personal behavioral patterns and determining the best coping strategies. But such data gathering (call it a check-in, if you'd like, since that can be compared to a medical checkup, which is as vital to your health as dealing with your stress properly) must be consistent for valid results.

One way to check in with yourself regularly is to start writing a journal. Take a few minutes each night to jot down your stressors and how you coped with them. This isn't an invitation to get negative and spill all the terrible about your day. This is simply a fact-gathering activity that you want to review later, so a list works great. Once a week, review your lists and notice what days were the most stressful. Look for consistent patterns such as, "I got up late and had to rush to work without breakfast." You may not even be aware how often something like this happens, and noticing it on paper helps you realize the problem, so you can address it proactively.

However, if you're not the journaling type, or just a little short on time, there is another option. I've put together a stress self-assessment worksheet to make analyzing your personal stress levels as simple and easy as possible. The worksheet consists of ten questions designed to quickly and accurately assess your stress levels. Answer the questions and follow the instructions to come up with your Stress Score. Take a few minutes to fill out the worksheet once a week, and you can track you scores over time, giving you powerful insight into your stress levels and how they are progressing.

You can download the free companion work-sheet on my website here:

https://www.bcfpublishing.com/stress-assessment

In addition to weekly check-ins, do a monthly check-in. Schedule it on your calendar so you don't forget. During your monthly check-in, notice whether your stress levels are going down (based on your weekly Stress Scores from the worksheet.) If you initially had a couple of weeks in the "50-70" range, for example, and now you're consistently scoring "80" or above, that's a great sign of progress. Notice what you did to help lower your stress. Conversely, if you're seeing an decrease in your Stress Score, then that also needs to be addressed. There's some advice on the worksheet, but in general you may want make sure you're following the exercises and strategies noted earlier.

Lastly, make sure to incorporate yearly check-ins into your mental health regimen. You want to make sure that you are reaching goals and sticking to plans of achieving everything you want. By reflecting on a year's time, you will see all the different changes you have experienced.

In the next chapter, I'll address dealing with challenges. Many people have a tendency to be overly critical of themselves and this only adds to one's stress level. Learning how to lessen that internal perfectionism is important to your mental health. Similarly, learning to notice patterns of excessive/obsessive worry and anxiety is important so you can then address the problem. Finally, I'll discuss how to avoid unhealthy coping habits such as those briefly mentioned earlier, including comfort eating.

5

Dealing with Challenges

"I don't run away from a challenge because I am afraid. Instead, I run towards it because the only way to escape fear is to trample it beneath your foot."

– Nadia Comaneci

You've now been through each of the steps necessary for dealing with stress in a healthy manner. You can identify the biological mechanisms that cause stress, which enables you to understand why, specifically, your body reacts to certain circumstances in a particular way. You know the different kinds of stress in your life. Furthermore, you have concrete strategies in place that you can draw upon when things get tough. Now it's time to finalize the stress relief roadmap you began in Chapter 1.

In this chapter, you will make a commitment that will help you finalize your plans for long-term success. Once you make a personal pledge, you'll be fully equipped to manage the various stressors that come your way.

This chapter will also give you further ideas for what to do if you run into trouble either in the short-term or an emergency situation. I'll discuss when and why it's important to seek professional help.

Finally, I'll provide you with additional resources you can draw upon such as stress groups, forums, online therapy possibilities, etc.

By the end of this chapter, you'll be ready to take on the world!

Keeping Stress Records

The most important tool to utilize throughout this journey is a record of your stress levels (as discussed at the end of the previous chapter). The more you know about your stress level, the better you can manage it. Keeping a consistent record is important for check-ins, but there are other benefits to this important step as well.

On days when you feel like nothing has changed, you can go back to the beginning to see how far you have actually come. Comparing and contrasting your progress is of great value. Furthermore, writing things down is a great way to make them come true. When you emphasize a certain goal or wish by jotting it down, you are already putting more energy toward it than anything else.

Do not stress over keeping these records, but try to stay strict with how much you track. You don't want to get to a point where you are worried and stressed because you forgot to keep a record, but don't be so relaxed with it that you can't even see the changes in your stress level.

CURBING PERFECTIONISM

Perfectionism can be deadly if you let it take you too far. Nobody is perfect, but we still tell ourselves we can be, and that we must be. Although we don't always expect those around us to be perfect, we still hold ourselves to this high standard, wanting more than anything to achieve a level of perfection.

If you learn to accept your own flaws, not only will you relieve stress, but you will also begin to love yourself much more. You realize how perfect you already are when you begin looking at the things that make you an individual.

You can still aim for success, just not for perfection. Know that there is no state of perfection, and the best possible state you can be in is the one that promotes continued growth and advancement.

Let's be clear: aiming for perfection in all areas of your life is setting yourself up for disappointment.

There's just too much to do on a daily basis to expect 100 percent perfection in every area—so don't. You're going to make mistakes. There will be slip-ups. Accept that inevitability and don't beat yourself up for it. It's normal. Constantly worrying about it is adds unnecessarily to your stress level.

Being Self-Critical

When people are critical, we most often react negatively. It's not pleasant when others—especially people we value in our lives—call out our particular flaws. But it's even worse when you're the one doing the criticizing because you may not even be aware you're doing it. Try a small experiment. Throughout the course of one day, keep a tally of how often you criticize yourself. Do you reprimand yourself because you rolled out of bed late? Note it. (No need to go into detail—just a few words like "missed my alarm" are enough.) Did your presentation not turn out the way you wanted, so you immediately start giving yourself all manner of negative feedback? Note it. At the end of the day, look at your list. Is it very long? When do you do the most negative self-talk?

Having identified your personal behavior pattern, you can now address a problem if it exists. What exactly is negative self-talk? Simply put, it's that constant negative head in your voice that puts you down, maybe even when you are doing positive things. No outside force is more powerful than your internal Negative Nelly, so it's vital you learn to identify it, so you can then retrain your mind.

I know someone who wears a small, discreet hair band around her wrist. Nobody knows it since women often wear such things. When she catches herself in the midst of negative self-talk, she lightly snaps the band. It doesn't sting like a rubber band, but it does provide a light physical reminder to stop the behavior. You need to develop a strategy to catch yourself because a constant barrage of internal negativity is as stressful as an external volley of criticism.

Psychologists suggest that one way to deal with negative self-talk is to give it a name. Any time that nagging voice starts up, you can firmly say, "Stop it, NAME." Some people choose humorous names, such as the afore-mentioned Negative Nelly. Whatever the moniker, the goal is the same. You want to call the voice out consistently and tell it to quit bugging you.

Another strategy for dealing with negative self-talk is to counter it immediately with something positive. So if you tell yourself, "I got out of bed late again"? Well, counter that with, "But I already had my clothes laid out, so I saved time." There's always something positive to counter a negative. It just takes practice and effort.

Once you learn to consistently identify negative self-talk and implement a plan for countering it, you'll be amazed at the results. People often react to the signals you're sending when you're not even aware of being negative, and they're likely to also react negatively. When you start being more positive in your feedback toward yourself, many times so will others.

Rumination

Ever heard of the term "ruminants"? It refers to animals like cows that chew their cud over and over again, reprocessing it to extract as many nutrients as possible. In human beings, "rumination" refers to obsessively focusing on a particular thought or problem. The difference between our rumination and a cow's is that a cow can get more out of its cud the second or third time around. Human beings can't necessarily do the same thing with a problem. Therefore, obsessing about something is psychologically "non-nutritive," if you will, as well as damaging.

Reflecting is fine, because reflection is productive. You're temporarily turning over a matter in your end, searching for a solution. When you find it, you move. When you ruminate, you stay stuck and can't move forward.

Rumination can be about things in the present, such as a mistake you made the previous day. Or you can ruminate about things that happened decades ago that embarrassed you. Regardless of when something occurred, if you mull over it nonstop, you're ruminating; and psychologists confirm that rumination can worsen conditions such as depression or anxiety, not to mention stress.

What can you do about rumination? As with negative self-talk, the first step is to identify it. Develop a personal strategy to catch yourself ruminating, such as a hairband around your wrist. Keep a tally for a day to identify when and why you ruminate. There may be particular triggers that you can isolate then avoid. For example, say you have a fear of speaking in public and have to do it frequently at work. You obsessively go back in your mind to that moment you messed up in a high school presentation, so the next time you have to present something at work, catch yourself when that automatic rumination begins. You know it's coming, so you can cut it off at the pass.

As with all kinds of stress, planning is the key to coping. So have a plan in place for rumination. Redirection is one strategy suggested by psychologists. As soon as you begin mulling over a particular thought like a sore tooth, turn on a favorite song. Sing along to it to redirect your thoughts. Or call a friend and talk about something totally unrelated to the rumination. Take a short walk down a new street and focus on observing everything around you in as much detail as possible. The goal is not to allow your thoughts to go down their usual path. Sometimes, by taking an actual, literal new route, you can jolt your mind into a new framework of thinking.

Meditation is also a proven strategy that helps with rumination because it involves letting go of your thoughts. If you're new to meditation, it won't be easy at first, but with practice, you'll be able to let your ruminations float away down the thought "stream" that many meditations reference that washes away anxiety and obsession.

Disappointment

Ever had a plan or dream and then failed to see it materialize exactly the way you, no matter how work you put in? That's inevitably disappointing. We all have grand goals that we want to see come to fruition. The problem is that those goals may not quite unfold in the exact fashion we hope, particularly if we're not being realistic.

For example, have you ever noticed that summer is right around the corner and decided you need to lose weight? Maybe it's the end of June and you determine that by the Fourth of July, you'll have lost fifteen pounds. That's probably not going to happen. So why set yourself up for the inevitable disappointment? Don't do that to yourself. Be realistic with your goals. And when you *are* realistic, and they don't pan out picture-perfect, that's okay. Maybe things turn out even better than you expected, even if they don't quite match the picture in your head.

Similarly, don't let other people disappoint you by having grand expectations that no one can fulfill.

Measure people by the same fair, reasonable standards you hope they'll hold you accountable for. Otherwise, you'll always be let down, time and time again, and that's a guaranteed stressor.

REDUCING ANXIETY

All of us feel anxiety at some point in our lives. While occasional anxiety is normal, and is even a biological safety feature programmed into all of us, similar to "fight or flight," it can morph into a disorder when it becomes obsessive. The American Psychological Association's definition of anxiety is "an emotion characterized by feelings of tension, worried thoughts and physical changes like increased blood pressure." Symptoms of generalized anxiety disorder include:

- Constant agitation
- Excessive worry
- Irritability
- Difficulty focusing
- Trouble falling asleep or staying awake

While there are many types of anxiety disorders, I'll focus broadly on two of the most common types: excessive worry and social anxiety.

Excessive Worrying

If you're constantly under stress, you're literally rewiring your neurological pathways to constantly worry. Think about the last time you were required to memorize something. How did you do it? Very likely, you repeated it over and over to yourself, whether out loud or by writing it down. And now, you will very likely always remember it, because it's ingrained.

Excessive worry has the same effect on your minds. Therefore, it's critical to retrain your brain to stop carving worry paths into it. As noted before, identifying stress is the first step to eliminating it, and that also applies to stress-generated worry. Develop a strategy to identify when you're obsessively worrying. Keep a tally for a day. Note particular triggers that you can avoid. Redirect your mind each time you find yourself worrying excessively. Have a plan ready so that whenever worry strikes, you know exactly what to do, whether it's watching a funny video, doing a crossword puzzle, talking with a friend, listening to music, etc. The goal is to send your thoughts down a different neural pathway from the one they've become accustomed to.

Social Anxiety

Social anxiety can cause a lot of stress. It is important to know the difference between just being nervous around others versus actually having social anxiety. We all get nervous on some level when meeting new people, especially if they have a high status, such as our boss or a political figure. Anyone might get scared on a first date. A person with social anxiety, however, will usually avoid these situations as much as possible because their level of nerves is so high that they have difficulty handling them.

Exposure and social practice are the most helpful tools to overcome social anxiety. Do not push yourself if it is too hard. Not everyone is going to be ready to confront social anxiety and might first need to start with the small things that stress them out.

If you constantly feel self-anxiety, the first step is to lessen it. To begin, accept the anxiety and stop condemning yourself for it. Some people are more anxious than others. According to Psychology Today, scientific research suggests that if your parents were chronically anxious individuals, you might also be. This doesn't mean you're forever sentenced to be anxious; it just means you may have a particular biological tendency toward anxiety.

Once you stop condemning yourself for being anxious—which in itself is breaking a vicious cycle because scolding yourself for worrying just adds to your stress—begin to replace common anxiety words such as "always" and "never." If you think, "I always mess up when I give a speech," replace it with, "I occasionally mess up. This doesn't mean it will help this time." Such words are anxiety triggers because they're so absolute. When you give yourself room to make mistakes, anxiety lessens. It takes practice and awareness to constantly catch yourself and rephrase your thoughts, but the long-term effects are tangible.

When you worry excessively, try using one of the breathing exercises highlighted earlier in this book. It will help you refocus your thoughts on something new. Similarly, anything else you can do to distract yourself is a positive step. Identify, accept, replace and redirect. That's a good game plan for dealing with excessive worry!

Medication

If your anxiety is something you're having trouble managing on your own, you might want to consider speaking to a professional and even taking medication. Talking to someone is always helpful, whether you are stressed, anxious, depressed or worse. While having friends and family around is great, you should also aim to seek out a professional who can give you an objective opinion, and one based in research and knowledge to help improve our mental stability at the core.

Some long-term effects of medication still need to be studied, but many people find that their lives change for the better after being prescribed something for their anxiety. Taking different drugs takes some getting used to, but they can help people who have no control over their mental illness finally take charge.

Individuals diagnosed with anxiety often need medication. However, before you consider going down that path, it's important to distinguish normal from stress-induced anxiety. The easiest way to tell the difference is to sit down and reflect on how your anxiety is impacting your life. While we all have times in our lives when we are anxious, most of us don't find that anxiety so overwhelming that it impedes our moving forward. A simple example is the fear of flying. Some people are nervous getting on a plane. That's normal anxiety. But when that nervousness has you worrying for weeks before the flight, and then you possibly can't even get on the plane, it's stress-induced anxiety on a level that needs intervention. Similarly, if you're so anxious about public speaking that it's affecting your work, that's not normal anxiety. If you can't go out and meet people because you're so anxious about any number of different scenarios, that's impacting your life, too, and should be addressed.

If, upon reflection, you find that anxiety is affecting you long-term, where you're anxious most of the time and it's is impacting your life decisions, consider seeking professional help. You may not need medication—therapy might be sufficient to help you cope with your stress. But if you do need medication, as indicated by a licensed professional, it's nothing to be ashamed of.

UNHEALTHY COPING HABITS

When stress becomes too much, we often reach for coping mechanisms that aren't necessarily healthy.

The only way to prevent this is to have one of the aforementioned stress-relief plans in place. Otherwise, you may fall prey to everything from self-harm and comfort eating to drug and alcohol abuse.

Self-Harm

When we think of self-harm, we might just picture someone cutting themselves. This is a common form of self-harm, but it is not the only way we hurt ourselves. If you are physically self-harming, such as cutting, starving, or hitting yourself or pulling out hair, you should seek professional help immediately. Don't feel ashamed. It is common among individuals with unmanaged stress.

Emotional Eating

Whether you overeat, starve yourself, or go through other forms of binging and purging, you have to look at the way you are eating to determine if it is healthy or not.

We stuff ourselves because we crave the release of good hormones in our brain that comes from eating. Sugary foods provide temporary "happy hormones" that make us feel good, but those feelings eventually fade, causing us to go back for more.

Sometimes, we starve ourselves because we do not like the way we look or we want to punish ourselves for something we did. Analyze your eating habits to determine if you are consuming food in a way that is hurting or helping you. The best way to figure this out is to assess how often you think about food. People with eating disorders ruminate on food to the point where it's all consuming. Do you tally calories constantly? Chastise yourself if you go over a certain amount of carbs? Make endless meal plans that involve repeatedly overhauling your pantry as you go from diet to diet?

Food shouldn't be the center of one's life. We eat to live. We shouldn't live to eat. If you're starving yourself, you'll always think about food because you are hungry. If you're binging, you'll still be thinking about it because you feel guilty. The bottom line is that if you're thinking of food more often than, say, wanting the occasional snack, or are vaguely considering what to prepare for dinner, your eating habits may be less than healthy and you may want to seek advice a dietician.

Substance Use

People sometimes use drugs, alcohol or tobacco to cope with chronic stress. While occasionally indulging in a drink or a cigarette is normal, drinking a six-pack by yourself, night after night, is a serious problem. This isn't a healthy way to cope with stress—it's destroying you physically, mentally and emotionally, even if you may not be able to see it because addiction is such a powerful force. Substance abuse of any kind generates its own kind of stress—and it can be lethal.

As for drugs, although the recreational use of marijuana is now legal in some parts of the country, it can also be unhealthy if it becomes a crutch for avoiding the real issue—your daily stress. Other drugs, such as cocaine or heroin, are highly addictive and have no positive effects whatsoever on stress level. If you are partaking in them, seek help immediately.

Conclusion

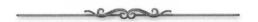

As we wrap up this book, my hope is that you're beginning the next chapter of your life with a new approach to stress management. Although stress is a universal, physiological response, people vary greatly in how they experience and cope with it. When I wrote this book, my intention was to provide you with a general understanding of stress. But I also wanted to guide you toward a personalized understanding of the stressors in your life and how you respond to them. I hope I've provided you with a diverse range of options you can use to cope better with stress.

I know I mentioned this before, but I think it's worth mentioning again: stress is not a negative thing. It's a biologically necessary response to perceived danger. The stress response is innate in the human body to protect us. That vitally necessary biological signal is trying to tell you something! Many times, we are so wrapped up in daily activities, meeting responsibilities and caring for others that we don't consciously acknowledge our stress signals.

Again, it's important to know the difference between stress that falls within normal limits and stress that is adverse to one's physical and psychological health. Remember, this is true whether you have a singular stressor or multiple areas of stress in your life. I know it's been said, but I can't emphasize enough the importance of knowing the cause of your chronic stress. If you find that your stress response to many or most situations is heightened, you can be sure there's an underlying cause. It could be rooted in your childhood. Many habits regarding stress management were developed in our formative years. As we become adults, we are challenged to adjust them according to our evolving needs and circumstances.

For those of you who have experienced a traumatic event or had a stressful childhood, there are a few key points I want you to take away from this book. If there is a repressed trauma in childhood that has not been dealt with, it is likely to manifest itself in a multitude of adverse ways. One of these ways is a heightened stress response and poor stress management. In this case, it's vital to revisit the trauma and the resulting emotions that have not been processed. This should be done with the help of a psychotherapist, a trained professional who can provide necessary support during the difficult or painful process.

It may be very painful to accept that you can never change who your caregivers were or what happened to you in the past. You have no control over that. But you do have control over how you respond to continuous stress. You may not believe it yet, but try to create an open space in your mind for the possibility that the future can be different from the past. While it's impossible for anyone to completely eliminate stress in life, it is possible to overcome chronic stress. It's within your ability to replace old, knee-jerk responses with new, healthier ones. Remember that as children, our reactions to stress are both learned and instinctive, but they are usually subconscious. Children have not yet matured enough to develop their own set of coping mechanisms that meet their individual needs. They rely on their caregivers to comfort and teach them how to comfort themselves. As children, sometimes our needs go largely unmet either because of abuse, neglect, or difficult, extenuating circumstances.

When this is the case, we may not feel supported at home and do not learn how to self-soothe as adults. The results are varied: we might look outside to fill the void and become co-dependent or addicted to harmful substances. We may internalize our negative experiences and isolate so extensively that our adult lives lack meaning and fulfilling relationships.

As I shared when introducing myself, one of my biggest obstacles was that I constantly looked for happiness and stress relief outside myself. I had not yet developed the tools I needed to rely on myself for comfort and stability. I would never have acknowledged it to myself, but I was depending solely on my husband, work, family and friends to make me happy. I avoided looking within to find out why it wasn't enough until I finally collapsed with exhaustion. Exhaustion can be a real, physical and psychological symptom of depression. For me, depression came from feeling so out of control that I no longer believed there was hope for me to feel happy and healthy again.

When you've reached this point, it's imperative to get help and start making changes right away. When I wrote this book, it was with people experiencing all levels of stress in mind. I also wanted to sound the alarm for people who are reaching a breaking point. Now that you have a base of knowledge, you can begin to make changes that will help prolong your life - and improve the quality of it, which is arguably the most important thing.

I had another wish for this book: to highlight the signs and symptoms of chronic stress so that you'll notice them before they completely take over your life. The effects of chronic stress usually worsen over time. They begin so innocuously that you hardly know it's happening (like the way it began for me). It could be the sudden emergence of daily headaches out of nowhere. Maybe you've seen your doctor, even gotten a second opinion, and they still seem unattributed to a physical cause. It may be that you feel happy with your career, relationship and life in general…yet, you're not quite enjoying the things you love and favorite activities the way you used to. You might be feeling tired and unmotivated, and the little things you used to take in stride now make you feel like screaming or lashing out. Anger is often telling us that something is wrong, and it's time to pinpoint what it is before the problem gets bigger.

Everyone has signs and symptoms. If this book has helped you recognize some of yours, or even helped you identify their cause, then I've accomplished one of my main goals.

AUTHOR'S NOTE

My other goal was to give you a wide range of mindful positive thoughts, behaviors and coping skills to replace the negative. Incorporating all five senses into meditation is an extremely helpful grounding force for me when I find myself at the start of a fight or flight reaction. It brings my focus into the here and now when I'm projecting fears into the future or obsessing about the past. Guided meditation also has a profound grounding effect for me. It centers me and helps realign my focus and clarity when they've gone haywire, which happens to us all at times. If it doesn't work right away; remember that this is normal. Meditation requires patience. Because most of us lead hectic lifestyles and are often inundated by stress, it can be exceedingly hard to surrender to the moment. If you've mastered your breathing and experienced a little bit of relaxation, you're off to an excellent start. If you're not able to completely let go of your worries for a moment but you can relegate them to the back of your conscious mind, then, again, the time was worthwhile. Meditation is one of those techniques that gets easier and better over time, so keep going.

There are times when I rely on avoidant behaviors and need to find a safe space to explore the past. Doing this provides me with insights about the present and sheds light on new possible solutions to the problems I'm facing.

We all have an inner child, but few of us have been taught to frequently check in on that smaller person, find out what she is feeling in response to past and current stress and comfort her the way you would comfort a child you encounter now. (If you are a parent, learn to treat your own inner child with the same gentleness and empathy with which you treat your son or daughter). You can start simply by repeating assurances and kind phrases in your mind. Eventually, your feelings and perceptions of yourself may shift from a place of demanding anger to love and acceptance. This strategy has been invaluable to me.

Just the other day, my computer crashed. I had stored all the notes for my next book on that computer, and I wasn't sure if I was going to be able to get them back. As if that wasn't bad enough, I was dealing with a health scare at the same time, and the results I needed to know hadn't come back yet. By the time I got home from work, I was already snow-balling and obscuring my usual logic. My thoughts raced, and I could feel my body reacting to the anxiety. My heart was beating faster, my legs were shaking, and I knew I was on my way to a full-blown panic attack. I felt as if I wanted to jump out of my body just to escape my mind.

The old Lauren would have allowed the panic to spiral out of control and snap like an animal at anyone who tried to help. After all, who could possibly understand the amount of stress I was under? But now I know that sweeping generalizations like this are the result of catastrophic thinking. Yet even after acknowledging this, I knew I still had to put a plan in place to deal with my anxiety. I mean, it wasn't going to melt away just because I realized it was there. Still, acknowledging felt like an act of kindness toward myself, and that alone had a calming effect.

I knew I wasn't ready to face my husband with my anxiety just yet. While I was still feeling so overwhelmed, there wasn't much anyone could say or do to help - and I didn't want to bite his head off like I used to during stressful days. So I pulled my car over and took some deep, calming breaths. As hard as it was to temporarily separate from my anxiety, I told myself that the problems would still be there if I give myself a break to regroup.

I chose a short meditative exercise. I tightened my hands into fists and then slowly let them go, feeling the tension drain out of them. Then I repeated this process with several other body parts that held a majority of my tension. Once I had finished this exercise, my circulation improved. I was thinking more clearly and was able to separate the three major problems in my mind. Tomorrow I would put aside enough money to get my computer fixed, and I'd just have to budget my daily expenses more tightly the next week. After all, my income is stable enough that I can compensate for surprise expenses, and that's something to feel proud of and thankful for. My attitude of gratitude led me back to my potential health problem, which was a big one. What if all of the things I had worked so hard to build were taken away?

Yet I didn't have any reason to believe it was true, and projecting into the future doesn't yield answers or outcomes; all it does is shatter your peace of mind in the moment. So, how could I relieve my anxiety before the test results came in? Still in a place of gratitude, I thought of my loving husband at home. Does he always respond in exactly the way I wish he would? No. But does he always make a sincere effort to understand me and give me what I need in the moment? The answer to that is a resounding, yes.

I started driving toward home. When I got there, I didn't snap at my husband or displace my anger by griping about our crowded kitchen space or the ingredients he forgot to buy when he did the shopping last week. I didn't do any of those things. The new Lauren, who is really just a healthier version of the old lovable one, took one last calming breath. Then she said, "You know, I'm really starting to freak out tonight. This week is just too much. Do you mind if we sit down and talk about it for a while?"

And guess what? His objective ear was more helpful than I thought it would be. (Okay, so maybe it always was). The point is, I'm glad I opened up. If I hadn't, I would never have had the chance to listen to my husband's outsider's perspective, which held insights I couldn't see from inside.

Guess what else? My test results turned out fine! (My computer is also alive and well, for anyone who is wondering). True, it could have gone the other way. Life is unpredictable; sometimes it changes in the blink of an eye. One of the hardest things we have to learn to grapple with is uncertainty. Life is full of beginnings and ends, and in many ways, permanency is an illusion. That's why it's so important to reach out and create a healthy support system and to be able to comfort ourselves as well. I wrote this book to help you achieve your own balance between external and internal happiness and reliance.

I want to end with an important reminder to put your health first and take excellent care of it. There is a symbiotic relationship between health and stress. In other words, stress affects your health, and your health affects your stress levels! That's one of the reasons why preventative healthcare is so essential. Serious illnesses have a major impact on quality of life, your ability to function, and your relationships. If you do have a serious or chronic illness, the importance of adequate stress management is underlined. It's even more important for you to reduce the harmful effects of stress. With illness or a metabolic imbalance, the body and mind connection is intensified and becomes even more vitally important. So, even if it means making adjustments that will affect others, do what you need to do to take care of *you!*

Set goals one by one and check them off as you go. Make sure they are realistic, and remember that no goals are too small if accomplishing them benefits you! If all checking a goal off your list does is make you smile in the moment, it's worth adding it. Your list of goals should be based holistically on your needs; it should address your body, mind and emotions. Healing from chronic stress is a long-term process, and not an overnight fix. The saying, "The journey is the destination" has become a tad clichéd, but it definitely applies here. Part of overcoming stress is learning to live in and value the moment. Perfection is not the goal; progress is. So if you've come part of the way but are still struggling, that's more than worth celebrating! Reward yourself with a relaxing day trip, a fun social outing or an enjoyable meal. Indulge in a new book or a movie night alone if downtime is what you crave. Even a long, hot bath can bring joy and relaxation.

Now that you have the tools, it's time to take your first step. I personally wish you the best of luck, but, more importantly, I want to remind you that healing is in your hands! If there's just one thing I hope you take away from my knowledge and experience, it's that you've already got all the tools within you. Now you just have to access and use them to your advantage. You've got this!

ADDITIONAL RESOURCES

Remember that you don't have to do this alone. Not only do medical professionals train for years just to help you and others with similar conditions, but there are free sources online you can access at any given time of the day. Never be afraid, ashamed, or embarrassed about reaching out for help. It is a brave thing to do and a great sign that you care about your health and safety.

Stress Groups

You might not have realized it, but there are many free support groups that meet regularly in your community. Many people have heard of AA, or Alcoholics Anonymous, but that is not the only support group available to help you overcome stress. There are groups that discuss different eating disorders, and help you to see whether you are overeating or suffering from anorexia and bulimia. There are other groups specifically targeted toward different types of trauma, whether from war or childhood.

Look to your area's community centers to see where people might be meeting and discover ways you can be part of a group that offers support.

Forums

Those who live in small areas or people with a debilitating social anxiety aren't always going to have what it takes to make it to a public stress support group. If you are not ready to get out there just yet, the internet is a great tool for endless forums, blog posts, and other discussion threads around a topic of your choice. Sometimes, if you are feeling especially anxious, you can even try Googling what to do. Don't let yourself forget how powerful that box in your pocket can be.

Online Therapy

While in-person therapy is certainly helpful, there are also many platforms online that offer therapy as well. This can even be done in addition to an in-person therapy session you already attend. Don't be afraid to reach out to online therapists, as they'll provide you with more help than you ever could have imagined.

Made in the USA
Columbia, SC
23 April 2020